THE REMARKABLE DEVELOPMENTS OF HEART AND CHEST SURGERY IN THE 20TH CENTURY

THE REMARKABLE DEVELOPMENTS OF HEART AND CHEST SURGERY IN THE 20TH CENTURY

ARMAND A. LEFEMINE MD

Copyright © 2015 by Armand A. Lefemine MD.

Library of Congress Control Number: 2014920737
ISBN: Hardcover   978-1-5035-1601-4
              Softcover   978-1-5035-1603-8
              eBook   978-1-5035-1602-1

All rights reserved. No part of this book may be reproduced or transmitted in any form or by any means, electronic or mechanical, including photocopying, recording, or by any information storage and retrieval system, without permission in writing from the copyright owner.

Any people depicted in stock imagery provided by Thinkstock are models, and such images are being used for illustrative purposes only.
Certain stock imagery © Thinkstock.

This book was printed in the United States of America.

Rev. date: 12/17/2014

To order additional copies of this book, contact:
Xlibris
1-888-795-4274
www.Xlibris.com
Orders@Xlibris.com
668573

TABLE OF CONTENTS

Prologue 9

    The Magnificent Development Of Surgery In The 20th Century 11
    New Book 11
    Anesthesia 12

Chapter 1 21
Chapter 2: Perspectives Of Thoracic Surgery 30

    Pediatric Cardiac Surgery 38
    Atrial And Ventricular Septal Defect 42

Chapter 3: Hypothermia 45

    Surgical Outcomes 58

Chapter 4: The Heart-Lung Machine 59
Chapter 5: Mininally Invasive Cardiac Surgery 65

    Types Of Valves 66
    Valve Replacement 66
    Perspectives Of Thoracic Surgery 66
    Valve Design 68
    Types Of Heart Valves 68
    Treatment Of Valvular Disease With Artificial Valves 69
    Mitral Valve Regurgitation 69
    TAVR Transventricular Aortic Valve Replacement 72
    Carpentier Mitral Valve 78

Chapter 6: Cardiac Arrhythmias, Surgical Treatment 80

Wolff Parkinson White Syndrome...85
Surgical Technique..88
Surgical Results...90
Postoperative Supraventricular Arrhythmias 93
Ventricular Tachyarrythmias...95
Ventricular Tachyarrythmias
Unrelated To Ischemic Heart Disease...96
Ventricular Tachyarrythmias
Associated With Ischemic Heart Disease................................. 101
Preoperative Electrphysiologic Evaluation.............................. 103
Surgical Indications And Contraindications 104
Intraoperative Mapping Procedure 105
Surgical Procedures 107

Chapter 7: Perspectives Of Thoracic Surgery................................. 115

Concept In PCI... 118
Percutaneous Coronary Intervention 118

Chapter 8: Chest Implanted LVAD 120

Coronary Assist Devices... 121
Chest Implanted LVAD..122

Chapter 9: Cardiac Interventions 124

Balloon Angioplasty..127
Coronary Angioplasty...128
Bypass Surgery Statistics...130
Mortality Rate Is Related To Age 132
Is The Patient Better?..134

Chapter 10: Heart Transplantation 136

Cardiopulmonary Homotransplantation 139
Lung Transplantation..140

    Types Of Lung Transplant 142

Chapter 11: Lung Transplantation...143
Chapter 12: Types Of Lung Transplant..146

    Assisted Circulation... 147
    Cardiac Asssist Devices 148
    Complications And Side Effects 154
    Chest Implanted Lvad 156
    Syncardia-Total Artificial Heart.. 157
    Home Discharge With Total Artificial Heart 158

Chapter 13: Lung Surgery-Tuberculosis And Cancer 160

    Lung Cancer 164
    Diagnostic Thoracoscopy 166
    The Trachea And Its Complications 167
    Lung Surgery 171

Chapter 14: Robotics..174
Chapter 15: Mediastinum 176

    Lymphoma...181
    Primary Extrgonadal Germ Cell Tumors Of The Mediastinum....182
    Cysts Of The Mediiastinum..182
    Enteric Cysts 183
    Pericardial Cysts..183

Chapter 16: Tumors Of The Esophagus 185

    Esophageal Carcinoma 185

Chapter 17: Barrett's Esophagus 190

    Aorta..191
    Dissecting Aneurysm Of The Aorta 198

Chapter 18: Chest Trauma 208

    Heart And Pericardium 212
    Tamponade 213
    Aorta Injury 213
    Esophagus 214

Chapter 19: Pulmonary Embolism 215

Epilogue 219
Achnowledgements 221
About The Author 223

PROLOGUE

THE FOLLOWING SERIES of discussions are what I consider to be an introduction to the world of thoracic surgery with special emphasis on cardiac surgery though on significant advances in all aspects of thoracic surgery. This is not to slight other areas that also experienced new additions and an impressive expansion of what could be accomplished by any specialty. I was fortunate enough to know and train with one of the pioneers in heart surgery and as a consequence met many of the renowned surgeons of the world at a meeting or at breakfast and though I did not always know the extent of their contribution and their place in history. I am privileged to have met them and to know them. It is hard even for me as a thoracic and a cardiac and a vascular surgeon by trade to fully appreciate the contributions of many of these men. Because of the state of thoracic surgery when they came along in the last 100 years it is not possible to appreciate what they did when they did it and the courage of the moment that changed surgery forever. There was a time when no one dared do anything with the heart no matter how disabling the problem. There was a time in the past century when no one dared to remove a diseased lung or esophagus because the mortality and morbidity was intolerable. There was a time when there were no antibiotics, parenteral nutrition, endotracheal tubes, anesthesia machines and even x-rays and it was a long time before we had cat scans, EKGs, and bottled anesthesia gases all of which we now take for granted. It is hard to appreciate the changes that ensued when the first surgeon stuck his finger in the heart to retrieve a foreign body, open a stenosed valve or swung down a subclavian artery to the pulmonary artery to pink up a blue baby. These were small steps in what has become a long series of new and dramatic series of operations that led to operations for all valves of the heart, lung resections, lung transplants, heart transplants, heart-lung transplants, resection and replacement of the esophagus, and a multitude of technical changes in the heart to correct dangerous and life-threatening arrhythmias.

The descriptions of what can be done now, which is extensive, is not accompanied with details of the surgical procedure. This not a textbook of how to do an operation. It is dedicated to acquaint you with what has developed in thoracic surgery in the 20th century. Certainly a list we can be proud of and even benefit from in the realm of pediatric malformations, to the aged and non-functional heart or replacement of all the valves of the heart and transplant a heart or a lung and even replace the heart with a mechanical heart. But what is of great interest to me and hopefully to you some picture of the pioneers and characters that made it all possible.

THE MAGNIFICENT DEVELOPMENT OF SURGERY IN THE 20TH CENTURY

NEW BOOK

This is the story of thoracic surgery in the 20th century. Though mankind has been involved with treating the sick, the invalids and the infirm for centuries there is nothing in the long story of medical and surgical treatment as impressive as the developments of the 20th century. There have been drugs natural and man- made as well as surgical procedures intended to correct or cure the life- threatening illnesses but nothing to compare with the giant strides in the development of drugs, surgical techniques and even the replacement of parts of the anatomy that have lost their natural and life sustaining function. The field of thoracic surgery has probably been the most exciting and revolutionary area to practice and work in the twentieth century. There have been many notable changes and advances in all areas of medicine and surgery but none so dramatic or exciting as has happened in thoracic surgery meaning surgery of the chest and all its contents to include such organs as the heart, lungs, great vessels (aorta and its branches, vena cava), esophagus, and trachea, as well as a complex lymph system and network. These organs and systems are the basis of life, health, nutrition, circulation, respiration, lymph, and general appearance. When normal anatomy and normal function are absent or altered to the abnormal or diseased by infection, metabolism, genetic inheritance or abnormalities resulting from the processes of pregnancy we have big problems to solve. Some cannot be solved or corrected and some die. There is risk in all surgery just as there is risk in doing nothing. Sometimes the congenital abnormality is diagnosed in utero and there is now some experience by some courageous surgeons to perform corrective surgery on the fetus in utero. This also requires a courageous patient. But the story of thoracic surgery is full of courageous surgeons and patients, new techniques, new inventive equipment to support an organ such as the heart or lung or even to replace these organs temporarily or permanently. We now have the ability not only to cure deadly infections in the lung but also to replace the diseased lung with a transplanted lung. It is the same with the heart. Artificial man-made vessels can replace some or all of the aorta and its branches if needed. Cancer of the lung, tuberculosis, cancer of the esophagus, mesothelioma of the pleura, and tumors of the heart all figured in the early story of chest surgery before the rush to fix the heart with all its complexities. It may be worthwhile to review some history of surgery and anesthesia to appreciate how we got here and where we came from. It is an intriguing story of what can happen when the right people with inventive fervor have the tools to work with as well as the ideas and the courage to develop them. With all the new knowledge and techniques of the past 70 years there have been monumental changes in the way medicine and surgery are practiced as well as how the doctors are compensated for their services. No longer does the general practitioner come to the home to deliver a baby or remove the tonsils or sew up a laceration. The doctor whether he be a generalist, an internist, or a surgeon or one of the many specialists that may have contact with a patient is threatened by malpractice suits that alter what he does and what he is willing to do. And that often includes delivering babies. The cost of medicine and medical care have skyrocketed and much of this is due to the development of medical insurance and governmental programs and managed care and the role that employers now play in the medical care picture. In looking at the development of thoracic surgery in the last 70 years we need to examine the important role that anesthesia played not just in the last 70 years but in history. Certainly without the development of general anesthesia, tracheal intubation and all the machinery to control anesthetic gases and oxygen in a safe effective manner there could not have been the operations we will talk about later. The same can be said for the development of antibiotics and the control or prevention of lethal infections and the cure of destructive infections such as tuberculosis.

ANESTHESIA

Early Arab writings mention anesthesia by inhalation. The history of surgery can be traced back to Arabic civilization even as early as the year 1000 AD when Albucasis described his achievements in laparotomy (opening the abdomen) and Caesarian section (delivering babies by opening the abdominal wall). This was at a time when there was little to offer in terms of pain relief or comfort during and after the procedure. The effective local anesthesia was cocaine later developed and used Karl Koller in eye surgery (at the suggestion of Sigmund Freud) 1884. A German Surgeon, August Bier, was the first to use cocaine for intrathecal (spinal) anesthesia. But the inhalational anesthetics really made it possible to do complex abdominal procedures as a routine much to the benefit of the patient with that precious relief of pain if you were lucky enough to be where the techniques and equipment and medical training made it possible. The idea of anesthesia by inhalation was the basis for the soporific sponge (sleep sponge) introduced by the Salerno School of Medicine in the late 12th century by Ugo Borgognoni (1180-1258) and in the 13th century. The sponge further described by his son was soaked in a dissolved solution of opium, mandragora, hemlock juice and other substances. The sponge was then dried and stored. Just before surgery the sponge was moistened and then held under the patient's nose. The fumes rendered the patient unconscious. In 1275 a Spanish physician, Raymond Lullus made a volatile flammable liquid called 'sweet vitriol'. This was one of the very first inhalational anesthetics used in surgery. In the 16th century a Swiss born physician commonly called Paracelsus made chickens breathe 'sweet vitriol and noted that they not only fell asleep but also felt no pain. Like Lullus before him he did not experiment on humans. In 1730 A German chemist, Frobenius, gave this liquid its present name' ether' but 112 years would pass before ether's anesthetic qualities were fully appreciated. In 1772 the English scientist, Joseph Priestly, discovered nitrous oxide but neither he nor a chemist Humphrey Davy pursued the matter as an anesthetic. An American physician, Crawford Long, noticed that his friends felt no pain when they injured themselves while staggering around under the influence of ether. A student had two small tumors removed on March 1842 under the influence of ether in a painless operation. Long did not announce his discovery until 1849. William Morton, a Boston dentist conducted the first demonstration of the inhalational anesthetic. Morton unaware of Long's work was invited to the Mass General Hospital to demonstrate his new technique for painless surgery. After Morton induced anesthesia John Collins Warren removed a tumor from the neck of Edward Gilbert Abbott. In a letter to Warren, Oliver

WendellHolmes proposed that the state induced should be termed 'anesthesia'. Morton at first attempted to hide the actual nature of his anesthetic substance and received a patent but the news spread quickly and by late 1846 surgeons in Europe including Liston, Diffenbach, Pirogov, and Syme quickly undertook numerous operations with ether.

Chloroform was discovered in 1831and the use of chloroform in anesthesia is linked to James Young Simpson who found chloroform's efficacy in 1847. Its use spread quickly and it was used on Queen Victoria during the birth of her son Prince Leopold. Chloroform is not as safe an agent as ether especially when administered by an untrained practitioner. Early on medical students, nurses and sometimes members of the public were pressed into giving anesthesia. This led to many deaths that otherwise could have been prevented. John Snow of London in 1848 published articles on "Narcotism by inhalation of vapours" in the London Medical Gazette. He also involved himself in the production of equipment needed for the administration of inhalational anesthetics. Chloroform was never in general use in the US but ether was the basic volatile anesthetic well into the 20th century. I can remember my appendectomy about 1940 that was done under ether anesthesia. It was not a bad experience except for the postoperative complications that were quite common then before the advent of antibiotics such as sulfanilamide and penicillin. A variety of fluorinated ethers have become available since that time. These are all administered by an anesthesiologist or anesthetist through an anesthesia mask, a laryngeal airway or tracheal tube connected to some type of anesthetic vaporizer and an anesthetic delivery system. The anesthetic agents that are now in use include isofluorane, desflurane, nitrous oxide, and servofluorane. The ideal volatile anesthetic has the property of being liquid at room temperature but evaporates easily for a smooth and reliable induction and easy maintenance of anesthesia with minimal effect on other organs. In addition it is odorless and easy to inhale and safe for all ages and pregnancy. Nitrous oxide even at 80% concentration does not produce surgical level of anesthesia. This brings us to the other items that made surgery safe and possible in the 20th century. The endotracheal tube now a commonly used instrument in anesthesia and emergency resuscitation is a flexible tube made of rubber or plastics with an inflatable balloon at its distal end so that the anesthesiologist has total control of the ventilation and the mix of gases and oxygen. It is hard to pinpoint the origin of this instrument but it is used routinely in general anesthesia. And because the placement of this tube is uncomfortable it is placed after the patient is unconscious from an intravenous barbiturate or an anesthetic gas.

One of the notable discoveries and addition to the field of surgery was the introduction and availability of the X-ray tube and the diagnostic possibilities for the heart and lungs. Roentgen published his first paper on the new rays he had discovered in 1895 and the course of medical history was forever changed. This was particularly true for chest surgery at a time when tuberculosis was a common and often a devastating problem in the lungs though it may affect other organs too. Wilhelm Roentgen was awarded the first Nobel prize in 1901. Of interest is the fact that he did not patent his discovery because he did not want to profit from it and he wished it available to all. The other almost simultaneous develpment in the early 20th century was the development of antibiotics for the treatment or prevention of infection. Three drugs became available almost simultaneously and were available by World War II These were penicillin, streptomycin and sulfonamide. There is no question that penicillin was the most important of these because it was effective against staphylococcus aureus commonly the cause of wound infections and lung infections and because it was effective against streptococcus which is causative of rheumatic fever and rheumatic heart disease which we will discuss in detail later. Streptomycin gained much respect and use because it was found effective against tuberculosis which was found to be relatively common and very infectious particularly amongst the poor and in crowded conditions. Tuberculosis became a chronic and very destructive infection in the lungs though these were not the only organs affected.

Thus anesthesia, antibiotics and x-ray were all available in the early 20th century which made possible the rather aggressive development of the techniques in chest surgery. The development of abdominal, orthopedic, neck surgeries, as well as gall bladder, stomach, intestines, and thyroid surgeries preceded the surgeries of the heart and lungs because the technical demands in the chest were greater as were the mortality and morbidity. In 1933 interest in chest surgery awakened when Edward Churchhill demonstrated that portions of the diseased lung could be safely removed and Evarts Graham performed the first successful pneumonectomy for cancer at a time when mortality rates were about 50% due to clumsy techniques and septic complications. In 1937 a blood bank is opened at Cook County Hospital for collection, donation, and preservation of as well as typing blood, an invaluable service for complicated surgical procedures. In 1938 a surgical resident at Boston Children's Hospital performed the first major operation on the great vessels of the heart by ligation of a patent ductus arteriosum. That surgeon was Robert E Gross who would go on to fame for a number of procedures in pediatric heart surgery.

World War II provided the setting for new thinking and especially for the courage to do things that some pioneers did because there was the opportunity and especially the necessity to do something that would not get done in ordinary time. Thus the 40s and early 50s saw attempts at saving lives and problems that would not ordinarily present themselves in the adult sphere and this was certainly true for adult heart surgery. A fine example of this is Dwight E Harken MD who as an Army surgeon began operating on the adult heart because there were soldiers with foreign bodies in their hearts that were accessible if you were willing to enter the interior of the heart, an area that was not to be invaded in the ordinary book of surgery. Dr. Harken operated on more than 130 soldier-patients removing bullets and shell fragments from great vessels, heart muscle, and heart chambers. This was in an era when most thoracic surgeons were unwilling to attempt any heart operation beyond repair of the pericardium. His training was at Bellevue hospital and later in an Academy of Medicine Fellowship in London where he specialized in Thoracic Surgery. Some of his work was a direct outgrowth of his work in Bellevue and London on bacterial endocarditis, a condition that was then incurable and 100% fatal. Dr. Harken believed that if you had a condition that was incurable and a rational concept of how to attack it you had a right to try and did create bacterial endocarditis in dogs but the war intervened and he was confronted by the reality of injured soldiers as a medical consultant in the European theatre. He convinced his superiors to allow him to perform elective heart surgery in these soldiers who would otherwise not survive. For the first time a surgeon actually handled the heart of a significant number of patients. He went where no one had gone before but private practice did not provide him with healthy heart surgery candidates. He did manage to perform his first successful valvuloplasty in June 1948. He was beaten by Charles

Bailey of Philadelphia by 4 days neither being aware of the others activity. We will deal with Charles Bailey's activities later in our studies

This was the setting for the century of cardiac and vascular surgery. The list of new surgical procedures in the chest and in particular the heart and great vessels cloud out similar interests in other countries such as England and Italy but this was a time of war and war creates disaster and opportunity for some trained surgeons in uniform such as my mentor and chief, Dwight Harken. It was the opportunity of a lifetime.

We might spend some time considering the state of the art of chest surgery when Dr Graham came on the scene at Barnes hospital in the years following World War I. Surgeons became interested in empyema, lung abscess, bronchiectasis, and tuberculosis. Cancer of the lung seems not to be a common finding and was considered a rare entity. Intra-thoracic operations were fraught with high mortality and morbidity unacceptable 50 years later. Only the dedicated and the brave surgeons would be willing to risk their reputations to the shocking mortality rates and septic complications associated with chest surgery. Tuberculosis was treated by collapse of the lung which was accomplished by inducing pneumothorax or by thoracoplasty (a term used to remove portions of ribs in order to collapse the chest wall and the lung beneath it). Surgery for lung abscess or bronchiectasis was managed by open drainage. (which usually meant removing a portion of chest wall for drainage.), cautery excision, or an attempt at lobectomy. Empyema was managed by catheter drainage or by rib resection or even by thoracoplasty. Thoracoplasty or removal of portions of ribs was a very disfiguring operation especially if it involved the whole chest wall on one side. In 1922 Lilienthal reported treating 31 cases of bronchiectasis by resection of lung tissue with a mortality of 42%. Seven of his 10 patients who underwent resection of more than a single lobe died. In Sauerbruch's Clinic 10 sequential lobectomy patients died before one patient survived. In Graham's 48 cases of bronchiectasis treated by lobectomy there were only eight successes. Lobectomy or the removal of a lobe of a lung was a formidable procedure though now we consider it as routine. There was still much to learn and techniques to develop. Plus antibiotics, blood banks and anatomical dissection were still to come. Lung abscess and bronchiectasis led to thin wasted individuals who had a chronic cough and putrid sputum. Finally Brunn of San Francisco described six one stage lobectomies for bronchiectasis with one death. The cuffed endotracheal tube for control of anesthesia was not reported until 1928 and endotracheal tubes for anesthesia were not generally accepted until that time. Ether and nitrous oxide administered by face mask were the anesthetic techniques of choice. The effects of open pneumothorax were still being debated and tolerated by the empyema commission. In 1935 Graham used his cautery technique on 76 patients with bronchiectasis with a mortality under 15%. The results for pneumonectomy for cancer were dismal world wide. By 1933 two patients in the world had survived a two stage pneumonectomy for bronchiectasis using a tight ligature around the hilum to create a sloughing lung that was removed two weeks later. This is rather primitive by today's standards but represents the development that the U.S. and others on the battle fields of world war I went through. A far cry from the meticulous dissection that is now standard. No patient had survived total pneumonectomy for cancer of the lung. On April 5th 1933 Graham took patient Gilmore to the operating room. Though a lobectomy was planned it was obvious that a pneumonectomy was required. After consultation with Dr. Chalfont, friend of the patient, a pneumonectomy was performed. A rubber catheter was placed around the hilum to constrict arterial and venous blood flow for 2 to 3 minutes and when no cardiovascular collapse occurred Dr. Graham removed the lung by dividing between the clamps and placed three sutures around the hilar stump. In order to obliterate what looked like a huge cavity he performed an eight rib thoracoplasty to allow the chest wall to collapse against the hilum. After the lung was removed the mucosa of the bronchus was cauterized as well as being treated with a 25% silver nitrate solution before being transfixed with a no. 2 chromic catgut suture. These technical details would now be considered primitive so unlike present day technique with its anatomical dissection without the disfiguring thoracoplasty or extensive removal of ribs. Radon seeds were introduced into the severed pedicle. A catheter drained the thoracic space to an underwater seal under the bed. The patient survived and returned to his medical practice. The first is hardly ever perfect and in this case hardly a model for the future but proved that pneumonectomy for cancer was possible. Following Gilmore's successful operation there were 16 consecutive failures. Three years elapsed before a second survivor appeared and Graham became known as the "Butcher of Barnes Hospital". But at the end of 3 years there were 5 cases in a row without a fatality. Graham went on to make great contributions to staff development and surgical education, the American Cancer Society, the American Board of Surgery, and a number of national and governmental committees. He was the Editor- in- chief of the Journal of Thoracic Surgery from its inception in 1931 to his death in 1957. Following the Graham pneumonectomy, Drs. Rienhoff at Johns Hopkins university and Archibald at McGill University described the technique of individual ligations of the hilar vessels and bronchus. Within a year controlled respiration using a cuffed endotracheal tube appeared, and antibiotics were available, (Prontosil, Sulfanilamide). Sodium pentothal induction was available instead of drop ether and dissection of the hilum was refined. General thoracic surgery of the lungs was about to enter another phase as antibiotics began to appear particularly streptomycin for the ravages of tuberculosis. Sterile techniques were refined and septic complications were reduced.

Even when I started my career in thoracic surgery in 1957 tuberculosis was the primary problem for the non-cardiac thoracic surgeon. Throughout the country there were whole hospitals devoted to the medical and surgical treatment of tuberculosis. I obtained a job as a surgeon in a VA hospital and was soon introduced to the complications of advanced tuberculosis of the lungs and the variety of surgical procedures available at that time. It was a demanding course in surgery of the chest as well as the treatment of an infectious disease and its destructive course in the body especially in the lungs. Tuberculosis could be a small nodule or it could cause destruction of a lobe or even a whole lung with calcification, empyema, purulent sputum, and abscess sometimes even involving the ribs. Treatment was always a challenge and required special judgement and knowledge. It was often accompanied by poor nutrition and depression that interfered with a normal life and active work. Fortunately at the time I faced these problems effective chemotherapy was available in the form of streptomycin which became available in 1944.

Tuberculosis has a long history dating back to the early Greeks. Morgagni popularized post mortem examinations and there followed an understanding of the disease process. During the 18th century it was recognized as a communicable disease. Famous people succumbed to the disease including Chopin, Keats, Chateaubriand. Spain and the small kingdoms of Italy recognized it as a communicable disease and enacted laws to prevent its spread. In France and Rome it was treated with dread and avoidance by servants and taxi drivers. Koch silenced the speculation. He identified the culpable organism and established it as a communicable disease. The x-ray of Roentgen established the means to a diagnosis. The Koch phenomenon or now known as the tuberculin test was the injection of a substance secreted by the tubercle bacillus or injection of the tubercle bacillus itself into the skin to gauge the reaction as a test that could be used to verify an infection or a prior infection. Prior to modern therapy the disease was regarded as uniformly fatal. Prolonged rest was regarded as the best treatment, thus the establishment of many sanatoria. History is replete with stories about attempts to treat this disease and most of them center around establishing sanatoria for rest therapy such as those written by John Hilton, Galen, Brehmer (Germany), and Trudeau (U.S.) all for the so called rest therapy, all in the 19th century. By 1946 Webb was able to report that there were 80 thousand cases in this country(U.S.). With the advent of anti-tubercular drugs the population of the sanatoria rapidly decreased and in 1954 the Trudeau Sanitorium closed its doors. There were a number of procedures that were used in attempts to drain empyema of the lung but these did not come into prominence until streptomycin became available. Up until that time the treatment of lung abscess short of going into the chest cavity and attempting resection of a lobe or the entire lung was indeed difficult.

CHAPTER 1

DIAGNOSTIC CARDIOLOGY WITH the use of catheters advanced to all chambers of the heart along with diagnostic radiology became a reality when Forsmann in 1929 initiated the catheterization process by passing a 4 French ureteral catheter into his own brachial vein and advanced it under fluoroscopy to his right atrium. Methods for pacing the heart in heart block and the development of pacemakers by Paul Zoll as well as defibrillators to restore a normal rhythm by Bernard Lown all set the stage for heart surgery at mid mid 20th century. Heparin was now available as an anticoagulant and would be one of the essentials for open-heart surgery and the heart-lung machine. In the late 1940s surgical development came from two directions, one was the attack on congenital surgical problems, and the other was a serious attention paid to the possibility of correcting or at least palliate mitral and aortic valvular heart disease usually of rheumatic origin (rheumatic fever).

World WarII provided the setting for new thinking and experience with a form of heart surgery that would not have been possible except for the wartime setting. A fine example of this is Dwight Harken who as an army surgeon began operating on the adult heart because there were soldiers with foreign bodies in their hearts that were accessible if you were willing to enter the interior of their hearts an area that was not to be invaded in the ordinary book of surgery. Dr. Harken operated on more than 130 soldier patients removing bullets and shell fragments from the great vessels, heart muscle and heart chambers. This was an era when thoracic surgeons were unwilling to attempt any heart operations beyond repair of the pericardium. His training was at Bellvue Hospital and later an Academy of medicine Fellowship in London where he specialized in Thoracic Surgery. Some of his works were a direct outgrowth of his work at Bellvue and in London on bacterial endocarditis, a condition that was then incurable and 100% fatal. Dr. Harken believed that if you had a condition that was incurable and a rational concept of how to attack it, you had a right to try. He did create bacterial endocarditis in dogs but the war intervened and he was confronted by the reality of injured soldiers as a consultant in the European Theatre. He convinced his superiors to allow him to perform elective heart surgery in these soldiers who might otherwise not survive. For the first time a surgeon actually handled the heart of a significant number of patients. He went where no one had gone before and he aroused great interest in heart surgery. Civilian practice did not provide him with healthy heart surgery candidates. He did manage to perform his first successful mitral valvuloplasty for mitral stenosis in June of 1948. Harken performed the operation by fracturing the mitral valve commissures with his finger introduced through the left atrial appendage. The first patient survived but subsequent operations performed on six desparatly ill patients were failures. This was devastating but he started again with only two of the next 15 patients dying and restored his career. He spent the next 22 years as chief of thoracic surgery at the Peter Bent Brigham hospital. (as it was called then). His successes won him many supporters and was the basis for a number of different techniques used successfully such as the bare finger fracture, the transventricular valvulotome or even a commissural knife. The arrival of the heart-lung machine shortly thereafter in 1953 transformed not only the the field of cardiac surgery but the thinking and opened up the possibilities of new operations and the possibility of prosthetic replacement which is the direction he took.

We should look at the results that Harken and his group were able to achieve with these initial early techniques because they are representative of what was accomplished and what many surgeons of the world were unable to offer these previously inoperable patients. We must remember that many of these patients had been sick for years, some in congestive heart failure, many if not most were in atrial fibrillation with enlarged hearts, and probably had clots in the left atrium, and always there was the danger of converting mitral stenosis to mitral insufficiency if the commissure broke badly or created an embolic episode from a highly calcific valve. Almost all patients were on digitalis and prophylactic quinidine as well as prophylactic penicillin. Prophylactic penicillin was always continued indefinitely as a prevention against more rheumatism since it is a progressive disease. Ellis, Harkin et al studying the first 2000 closed valvuloplasties indicated that the operative mortality rate in group 3 (less sick) was below 1% and in group 4 was approximately 17%. At this time in history these figures were quite acceptable. In a subsequent study of 1817 patients with minimum followup of 5 years and spanning 16 years they assessed such factors as age, rhythm, mitral valve calcification and mitral insufficiency. The most striking difference in operative mortality was between group 3 and group 4 in the under 60 age group. The operative mortality was considerably higher in patients with atrial fibrillation than patients with sinus rhythm. The mortality rate was also higher in patients with 2 or 3 + mitral insufficiency compared with those that had O or 1+ insufficiency and in patients with 2 to 4+ valvular calcification. Ellis found significant improvement in 85% of group 3 patients at the end of 1 year. This was reduced to 66% at the end of 5 years. There are mounds of statistics associated with the development and application of techniques to mitral stenosis as the really first treatable heart valve and we will try to give credit for contributions as we proceed however there is one historical character that we must discuss because he earned a place and a reputation in cardiac surgery that is not only historical but interesting.

Charles P Bailey was born in New Jersey and was a cardiac surgeon that belongs to the post war group of surgeons that changed the world of surgery especially in the area of heart surgery. He practiced and made his reputation as an aggressive innovative surgeon in Philadelphia principally at the Hahnemann Hospital. He is credited with the first finger fracture of the mitral valve for mitral stenosis as well as a number of other techniques in the treatment of mitral stenosis. He was well known for his aggressive approaches to the heart and for his courage in attempting to correct mitral valve disease. He is sometimes referred to as wild Bill as he approached the mitral valve from a number of directions and developed a number of instruments that could be used through the atrium or through the apex of the left ventricle and positioned the patient for an approach in the right and left lateral as well as the facedown position. Dr Harken was long credited as the first to correct mitral stenosis because he published his success first but it was later proven that Bailey performed his first successful mitral commissurotomy as he preferred to call it 4 days before Dr Harken did his first valvuloplasty as he preferred to call the operation. Dwight Harken and Charles Bailey spent the next 20 years competing and sometimes arguing while they both developed technique and instruments that could be used through the atrial appendage or the apex of the left ventricle. They both did their first successful mitral valvuloplasty or mitral commissurotomy, depending on which one you talked to, in 1948 but the exact dates of the first successful mitral valve operation remained a mystery for years. There is little doubt that Harken published his operation in the medical literature before Bailey did and thus was the basis for his claim to priority. However many years later some adventurer found and stole the record of Harken's first success and proved that Bailey preceded Harkin by 4 days. Of course both deserve credit for monumental contributions to the development of heart surgery and certainly contributed mightily to the lore and the passion that attended the competition of two mighty personalities. I was with Harken a number of years and I met Charlie Bailey a number of times at surgical meetings where both men would have heated discussions about the best way to do certain things. After having conquered the mitral valve both turned their attention to the aortic valve and contributed to successful treatment and techniques for the aortic valve which in reality was a more difficult valve to treat surgically because it did not lend itself to a closed approach as easily or effectively as the mitral valve. With the mitral valve there was the atrial appendage through which the surgeon could insert his finger or an instrument to manipulate the valve and to separate the fused leaflets in the case of stenosis or stenosis with mild insufficiency. In the case of the aortic valve there is no appendage that could be used to insert a finger or an instrument with control in a high pressure vessel. Some surgeons including Bailey attempted to approach the aortic valve by sewing a vascular graft onto the side of the ascending aorta as a passageway to the valve for finger manipulation or even an instrument with intent to open the commissures of a diseased or sometimes destroyed valve due to intense calcification or a combined stenosis and insufficiency. A British surgeon Ross about this time contributed a technique and an instrument for use through the apex of the left ventricle for performance of an aortic valve dilatation for aortic stenosis. An addendum to the story of Charles Bailey: eventually retired from the practice of surgery to become a lawyer which he practiced in his later years.

 The aortic valve along with the mitral valve has historically cause the most fervor and attempts at surgical correction. Aortic stenosis like mitral stenosis is a very debilitating condition with almost complete obstruction of the outlet of the heart. Reduced exercise tolerance, congestive heart failure, enlarged heart, rhythm abnormalities, and clotting complications in the atria as well as calcification that usually destroyed the valve and even involved the bundle of His (arrhythmia problems) with heart block or abnormal rhythms. Hufnagel who was a contemporary of Harken provided an impetus to the use of an artificial valve when he designed and used a ball for placement in the thoracic aorta in patients with aortic insufficiency. He used it once but never repeated the procedure. This is where we encounter the thinking of Dr. Harkin who with the aid and help of a clever engineer named Cliff Birtwell found the ball valve design the answer to designing and manufacturing an artificial valve for replacing the highly diseased aortic valve. This of course was after the introduction of the heart-lung machine and the new reality of direct vision surgery inside the heart and aorta. This valve had a stainless steel base and a stainless steel cage with a silastic ball in the cage. There have been a number of attempts by other surgeons dating back to 1958 when Muller reconstructed a resected aortic valve using a tricuspid prosthesis made of Teflon cloth. In 1960 Harkin implanted the first subcoronary ball valve. Roe et al used a moulded tricuspid Silastc valve in the subcoronary area. The ball valve has been accepted as the standard for aortic valve prosthetic replacement until recent times. About this same time Starr working with Edwards Lab produced a similar ball valve that originally was intended for mitral valve replacement but soon found a market as a prosthesis for the aortic valve. Pirie et al stated that more than 10,000 Starr Edwards aortic ball valves were sold from 1962-1965. Extensive testing at many centers after implantation in humans attests to the durability of the silastic ball and the inertness of the stainless steel. The first successful ball valve placed in March 1960 had to be replaced in 3 and ½ years because of a parabasilar leak and there was no sign of wear or corrosion. There was some loss of mass in the ball. Biodegradation of the ball and malfunction was noted in a small number of the early series of Starr-Edwards ball valves. In 1963 Ross reported his early results with subcoronary homograft aortic valve transplants using freeze-dried formalin fixed and frozen valves. Barret-Boyes subsequently reported an extensive and very successful experience with freeze-dried homograft valves in aortic stenosis and aortic insufficiency. Present trend is to use frame-mounted heterologous valves (animal valves) or the tilting disc valve introduced by Bjork. The techniques of implantation are all similar using heart-lung bypass with or without cardiac arrest and possibly using coronary perfusion and hypothermia. Changes in the design of the original ball valve have included a prosthetic cloth covering for the struts and the base because of incidents of clot embolus. The theory is that the cloth will induce the development of a smooth endothelial like lining that will resist clot formation. Meticulous removal of all calcific deposits is often necessary. The insertion of a homograft valve without prior fixation on a stent requires some special technique. The aorta is opened with a long oblique incision carried down to the base of the non-coronary cusp. If the cusps are not calcified they are resected downto a 5mm. rim and the aortic root is measured by an obturator. The lower margin of the graft is trimmed to within 3 mm. of the rim. Three key sutures are placed at the commissural areas of the patient and the graft. In the Barret-Boyes technique a large remnant of aortic wall is used allowing a double line of fixation to the base of the aorta.

Reports of results (mortality) doing aortic valve replacement with the Starr-Edwards valve varied from 1.4% to 10.8% with an average of 5%. This includes both cloth covered and non-cloth covered valves. Bjork reported a 5 year experience in 470 patients with an operative mortality of 5%. Kay reported an operative mortality of 3% using the Kay-Suzuki disc valve. Statistics at the second national prosthetic heart valve conference in a review of 3620 cases, most of which were caged ball valve type, the operative mortality rate for the aortic valve was 15%, the late mortality was 10%, and the complication rate was 20%. The cumulative mortality was approximately 29% in 5 years. The results become more significant when in the light of the natural history of aortic stenosis. Retrospective studies have shown that within 2 years of the advent of symptoms of angina, syncope, atrial fibrillation, or left ventricular failure 50% of the patients are dead. Fewer han 25% survive 5 years after the onset of symptoms. The presence of congestive heart failure and atrial fibrillation is particularly ominous. With survival possibly limited to months sudden death may occur in as many as 24% of the patients. Data for combined aortic stenosis suggest that the progmosis is similar. For aortic insufficiency the prognosis is again related to the degree of symptoms and disability. If right heart failure is present the mortality approaches 85 to 100%. Sudden death in aortic insufficiency is common. Survival varies with the valve model. The greatest attrition occurs during the first 12 to 18 months after operation but after this period the life curves assume a more normal appearance. Bloodwell using a variety of caged ball valves found a cumulative mortality rate of 26% after 7 years followup. The cause of the late deaths included myocardial failure, coronary isufficiency, arrhythmia, thromboembolism, mechanical failure of the prosthesis, bacterial endocarditis, and cerebral vascular accidents. Over 2/3 of the patients surviving were free of symptoms.

Thromboembolism has been the most common complication of prosthetic valves and this has ranged from from 3.9% to 24%. With good anticoagulation this can be held to about 10%. Braunwald reported on thromboembolism in a series of 22 patients for over 22 months using the Brown Cutter ball valve which has a cloth covered cage and a silastic poppet. Mild hemolytic anemias are more common with cloth covered valves. Small orifices, metal to metal contact, turbulent flow, and even a diastolic murmur indicating some insufficiency have all been mentioned as causes. Postoperative endocarditis was a rare occurrence with adequate antibiotic coverage, though staphylococcus and even fungus organisms have been mentioned. Replacement efforts have been made and been successful but mortality is high. The most common fungus mentioned is Candida. However aspergilla and coccidiodes among others have been mentioned. The place for heterograft valves is yet to be determined and are mentioned for completeness. Obviously animal valves would be an advantage but technical problems associated with preservation techniques, late results and sources need refining.

The tricuspid valve does occasionally cause problems. It is usually combined with problems at other valves rarely as an isolated problem. It is the least common of the rheumatic valve problems. It occurs in 20-30 percent of patients with rheumatic mitral disease. Starr estimated that 28% of 464 patients had tricuspid disease at the time of mitral valve replacement and approximately half required tricuspid valve replacement. So it can be a serious complication. The pathology is similar to that of mitral valve disease such as fusion at commissures, thickening of leaflets, shortening of chordae and calcification. There may be complete stenosis or complete incompetence. The clinical picture may include pulmonary hypertension and fibrosis, a pulsatile liver, and peripheral edema. The clinical diagnosis is not difficult because the clinical manifestation is more obvious such as distended veins and pulsatile liver. The catheterization findings are elevated right atrial and end-diastolic pressure as well as elevated pulmonary artery pressure and characteristic angiography findings. The angiography findings are subject to being false findings because of the catheter lying across the valve. Atrial fibrillation may make interpretations difficult. The most accurate evaluation is with the finger at the time of operation. A low cardiac index emphasizes the need for correction. Minor degrees of insufficiency are well tolerated. The findings may be similar to mitral stenosis. The selection of an operative procedure may be difficult but usually amounts to annuloplasty versus replacement. Some surgeons have reported satisfactory results with plication of the annulus. Techniques of annyloplasty by Carpentier and deVega may be suitable when the regurgitation is functional but otherwise normal. Organic disease of the valve with stenosis and/or insufficiency may require replacement of the valve. Carpentier has introduced the concept of a fabric covered ring moulded to the annulus as a form of annuloplasty. He has evolved six sizes for adults and children and even smaller sizes for infants. Orifice size is determined by an obturator. Carpentier has reported the results in 150 patients. All of these patients had either mitral and tricuspid disease or triple valve problems. Hospital mortality in the double valve group was 9.5%. In the triple valve disease group the hospital mortality was 14%. Hemodynamic evaluation by catheter evaluation 1 year after surgery revealed normal valve function or minimal regurgitation. The deVega annuloplasty is a variation on the theme of a reduction in the size of the tricuspid annulus. It will supplant valve replacement in many institutions. It is designed to shorten the annulus by multiple stitches as the base of the mural leaflet to restore competence of the incompetent valve as long as the disease does not involve the septal leaflet to a size allowing two fingers in the orifice by tying each end of a purse string over a square Teflon felt. Annuloplasty by obliteration of the posterior leaflet has been favored by a number of groups. Kay used the technique for 14 years in 87 patients and reported an early mortality of 16% and a late mortality of 9%. Twelve were unsuccessful all because of the mitral valve repair or replacement. 53 patients had a good result in a follow up from 1 to 14 years. Pluth and Ellis reviewed their experience with 174 cases of tricuspid insufficiency associated with mitral valve disease treated with annular plication and with valve replacement in 37 patients. The hospital mortality rate was 31% for annuloplasty and and 27% for valve replacement. The most common reason for failure to survive was progressive tricuspid insufficiency and low cardiac output. More of these patients are in NYHA class IV. Survivors with tricuspid annuloplasty had less improvement than those with valve replacement. The incidence of late death was also highest in the group with annuloplasty. The proper treatment remains unsettled.

Bailey and Harken each had the stuff to persevere under trying circumstances. I doubt that either of them ever appreciated being grouped with the other, but they were constantly on programs together and criticizing each other's published and presented work. They were serious rivals who together opened up the field of valvular heart surgery.

There were a number of similarities between these two men. They were born in the same year, they died in the same year, and they were of an identical age (38 years) when they did their first successful valve operation. When they first reported a series of procedures they used the same format, which was to give the case history of each patient documenting all the viscissitudes: the torn appendages, the ventricular fibrillations, the rigidly calcified valves that resisted any surgical treatment. Having detailed each patient's course they subclassified the patients into those who actually had undergone the intended procedure. This allowed them to make more optimistic summaries than they otherwise might have. Who would blame them for this after all they had been through? And, of course, their optimistic forecasts were accurate. They knew how much they had learned in those first few operations.

Neither of them were full members of the surgical establishment. Hahnemann had been a homeopathic hospital and was not looked upon at that time as being in the same league as the other four Philadelphia medical schools. Dwight Harken certainly had an establishment base at the Peter Bent Brigham but, like Charles Bailey's procedures, those early operations were done at a number of community hospitals (Bailey's first five operations were done in at least four hospitals and Harken's in three). Harken never had the image of being a member of the Harvard hierarchy. Each of these pioneers followed his own path. The development of closed heart surgery was an entirely personal accomplishment by these two men.

Strangely, neither of them was elected to membership in the prestigious American Surgical Association, into which the leaders of American surgery are customarily received. Both were reviewed and rejected on several occasions. Harken, however, gave an invited lecture on mitral valvuloplasty before that body in 1951.

CHAPTER 2

Perspectives Of Thoracic Surgery

THERE IS INCREASING awareness of the discrepancy between the pathologic findings and the presence of heart block. Fibrosis localized to the conduction bundle unrelated to vascular disease is a common finding. Rheumatic valvular disease found in 5% to 10% of the patients with complete or high grade heart block is almost always aortic valvular disease with calcific invasion of the adjacent septum. Penton et al reported the presence of heart block in 12 patients with mitral valve disease. Luetic heart disease, congenital defects, the residua of diphtheria, lupus erythematosus, sarcoidosis, uremia, Chagas disease, and familial cardiomyopathy are other causes. Digitalis intoxication may be a precipitating cause in the development of Stokes-Adams Disease in patients with atrial fibrillation and associated partial or complete heart block. Digitalis can depress impulse initiation, prevent conduction through the atrioventricular node, cause paroxysmal tachycardia and produce ventricular fibrillation. The reported incidence of temporary heart block in acute myocardial infarction is significant as high as 25% in some series. Heart block arising in the acute phase of a myocardial infarction is significant. Heart block arising in the acute phase of a myocardial infarction rarely becomes a chronic problem requiring implantation of a pacemaker the conduction defect disappears in one or two weeks. In these cases pathologic studies have revealed only minimal lesions of the conduction system. There may be a need for temporary pacing in some patients and there may be a need for a permanent implantation of a battery run pacemaker in others. Statistics indicate that anterior myocardial infarction with aberrant types of QRS conduction is associated with a high mortality, the result of atrioventricular block. Heart block following operations for congenital or acquired heart disease is related to injury to the conduction system. This may be related to injury to the conduction system by suture, hemorrhage or necrosis. Injury may result in evanescent, temporary or, complete heart block. Hemorrhages, some with necrosis as a result of a suture passing through the bundle, encircling the bundle or in the vicinity of the bundle and are most apt to occur following closure of ventricular septal defects. Refinements of suturing technique have reduced this to less than 1%. Complete heart block following replacement of the aortic valve have been frequent. In some series although half were of a transitory nature. Severe calcific aortic stenosis with calcification invading or penetrating the annulus is the common factor in these. Sutures placed at the lower most portion of the non-coronary cusp were found to penetrate the entire thickness of the of the atrial wall in the region of the bundle of his. Clinical Course poses the danger of sudden death. Heart failure, dyspnea and angina are related. Syncope is the result of transient reduction or sudden interruption of circulation. The convulsions of a true Stokes-Adams attack result from more prolonged episodes of asystole or the arrhythmias of ventricular fibrillation and ventricular tachycardia. They need to be differentiated from those of carotid vessel occlusion and intracerebral vascular disease. Carotid vessel occlusion and intracerebral disease are more likely to manifest unilateral blindness and muscle weakness rather than syncope as in bradycardia or asystole. Data on survival after the onset of complete heart block vary but Friedberg et al found that 50% of a group of 100 patients were dead within a year of onset. Lawrence et al in a review of 49 patients with complete heart block secondary to arteriosclerotic disease followed over a 20 year period found that the majority were in the sixth and seventh decades of life. Twenty per cent died suddenly. Nine patients lived with restriction of activity from nine to fourteen years after onset. Nearly all a had persistence of heart failure or hypertension. Obviously there was a pressing need to develop a means of pacing the heart both in cardiology in general especially in cardiac surgery as it developed. Development of the implantable pacemaker which has become a standard and sophisticated instrument has progressed from single wire electrodes advanced through an arm vein to the right ventricle from an external battery pack or electric stimulater to implantable units connected to the heart usually the left ventricle directly from an implanted unit in the upper abdominal wall or an electrode to the right ventricle from a battery unit in the right upper chest wall. Both unipolar or bipolar catheters can be used. A variety of pacing modes are available, from asynchronous to synchronous to demand pacing when the rhythm is intermittent and unreliable. The most recent pacemakers will not only provide pacing in a synchronous fashion but will defibrillate the heart should asystole occur. These are marvelous bits of electronics and are a far cry from the original implanted pacemaker first used by Paul Zoll in 1952. Occasionally temporary wires are attached to the right atrial appendage if there is a danger of heart block after surgery because of the technique or the location of the bundle or the proximity of the sutures. If some form of heart block occurs or there is a danger of developing heart block postop the patient can be paced and the pacing wire can be removed without having to enter the chest when the danger of heart block has passed. Atrioventricular synchronous pacers are available for whom the atrial contribution is important and for whom the atrium provides a means of adjusting ventricular rate to the to the requirements of stress. An atrioventricular sequential demand pacemaker consists of two stimulating catheters one atrial and one ventricular. Both stimulators are recycled by sensing a ventricular R wave. The atrial electrode only stimulates and the ventricular electrode serves as a sensor as well as a stimulator. The mechanism is such that the pacemaker may remain dormant or may function as a preset pacer, or may stimulate both atria and ventricles in synchrony. Other designs allow sensing of the atrial impulse with a 390-msec delay to simulate a normal atrioventricular sequence. There are unipolar and bipolar catheters available. A bipolar catheter has both cathode and anode at the tip of the catheter approximately 1 cm apart. A large variety of permanent pacemakers is available. Batteries have a different life-span, the most recent one is the lithium iodide with functional lives of 10 to 20 years. I think it is safe to say that all these mechanical and electrical gadgets and parts replacement represent gigantic advancements in the ability of cardiac surgery as a science and a life- saving modality. In a short span of time cardiac surgeons with the ingenious help of industry and the persistent efforts of laboratory teams both surgical and medical have achieved a phenomenal array of techniques, and replacement parts along with the mechanical and electrical apparatus to support concepts of repair, reconstruction, restitution of function, and even replacement of whole organs such as the heart, lungs, and major vessels, such as the aorta or the coronary arteries, pieces of organs such as valves, and even walls of the heart that were partially destroyed by tumor or injury. New valves both mechanical and, new designs, utilizing balls or discs as well autologous, homologous, and heterologous valves with and without supporting frames were introduced almost without much interruption during this period. Methods for preserving heart function such as cold, special solutions and additives for the coronary blood when the coronaries were perfused were common. Heart valves were preserved in special solutions to prevent rejection by the body. The energy devoted to preserve cadaveric valves as well as develop new designs has been the interest of many men in many countries especially the US and Great Britain. The development of new techniques and new valves is well illustrated by the current interest and application called TAVR or transarterial or even transmyocardial placement of an aortic valve that is at the end of a catheter device and then unfolded or allowed to expand in the anatomical location. This is certainly a marvelous technical feat, one that can be done without opening the chest or in certain cases at least without opening the heart or aorta. The mortality of aortic stenosis or combined aortic stenosis and insufficiency left untreated when symptomatic can be quite high. A design was introduced for the mitral valve replacement. The designs were amazingly similar. They were ball valves with hollow metal balls in a metal usually cloth covered cage. There is a story for the cloth covering because it was soon noticed that though they functioned well and did the job they were prone to develop clot and produce a certain percentage of embolization and possible serious complications. The cloth covering the base and struts was used to develop a clot resisting surface that worked amazingly well.

The story of the replacement valves of the heart is long and complicated if done in its entirety and certainly is a tribute to the courage as well as the ingenuity of the men working in this field. There were deaths and complications as might be expected in a group of patients with some very complicated lesions, some close to death, some with associated lesions, some with multiple lesions requiring multiple valves and many with other types of disease affecting the heart such as coronary artery disease. The cloth-covered valves however showed a markedly reduced incidence of thromboembolism even without anticoagulation. The incidence of thromboembolism without anticoagulation can be reduced to 1% with this design. This of course can be a great advantage to those who cannot tolerate any form of anticoagulation. Systolic gradients do vary with the size of the valve which is dictated by orifice opening. The disc valve with cage has also received extensive trial on the premise that it produces more favorable hemodynamics with a larger frustrum area but this has not proven to be true. Valves with silastic or Teflon discs have shown a significant incidence of wear which restricts their use. The tilting disc valve originally introduced by Wada was subsequently redesigned by and imtroduced by Bjork in 1969. It has the advantage of a very low profile, a central flow concept, free floating lens without a cage and an extremely favorable ratio of inlet orifice and to mounting ring. As a result this valve has excellent hemodynamic function in smaller sizes. Peak systolic pressure and gradients across an aortic may vary depending on size and also on the location and design. It averaged 12.5 mm for the Bjork-Shiley, 17.5mm for the Starr Edwards and 27mm for the Kay-Shiley. Gradients become important for small aortic roots. The unstented homograft valves may present the best hemodynamics. Mortality rates are always significant information however there are so many variables in any one group that it is hard information to evaluate. Early mortality for the Starr-Edwards prosthesis for a variety of reports from the literature varied from 1.4to 10.8% and late mortality varied from 2.3 to 24 per cent. The greatest attrition happens during the first 12 to 18 months after operation. After that the course is more normal. In 1969 Bloodwell reported using a variety of caged ball valves in his long-term patients with a cumulative mortality of 26% after 7 years of followup. The problems that arose were myocardial failure, coronary insufficiency, arrhythmia, thromboembolism, early and late deaths were usually the result of myocardial failure, coronary insufficiency, arrhythmias, thrombo- embolism, mechanical failure of the prosthesis, bacterial endocarditis, and cerebrovascular accidents. This is all a simplified look at the success and failure with one valve but similar problems arose with the other valves. However we must give credit to these early pioneers who paved the way, and showed that it could be done in an era of time when there was nothing to offer but hope and well wishes.

But there is even more. Though the valves could now be replaced using an open heart machine with all its complicated aspects many patients were not eligible because of age, poor condition and other problems such as intolerance of drugs, previous surgery etc. There arose a new technique that is finding its way into the lexicon and the dictionary of new procedures and it is called transcatheter aortic valve replacement. Aortic valve disease is commonly treated now by aortic valve replacement but the open procedure is considererd dangerous for high- risk patients with multiple organ dysfunction. Approximately 30% to 40% of elderly patients with severe, symptomatic aortic valve stenosis are deemed ineligible because of high perioperative risk. Transcatheter aortic valve replacement has been developed as an alternative technique for just such a group. The conventional surgery is not an option for patients of advanced age. If left untreated aortic stenosis is a rapidly progressive disease with a mortality of approximately 50% in the first 2 years. Approximately 30-40% of elderly patients with severe symptomatic valve stenosis are deemed ineligible for surgery because of high perioperative risk. However the introduction of a percutaneous approach by Cribier in 2002 followed by a refinement to a transfemoral approach by Webb and associates in 2005, has challenged the idea that these high risk patients are inoperable. Trans femoral [TAVR] is the only therapy that has been associated in a randomized trial with survival rates equivalent or superior to those of surgical experience in Euorpe. In elderly patients the aortic valve as well as the aorta is often heavily calcified and brittle which pose a risk because manipulation often dislodges calcium and may cause a stroke. TAVI is less invasive and offers a lower mortality risk. The true stroke risk is still being evaluated. Kneitz et al reported a case of a 90 year woman diagnosed with severe aortic stenosis aggravated by physical activity. She had a history of hypertension, chronic obstructive disease, hypothyroidism, congestive heart-failure, atrial fibrillation and renal insufficiency. She had undergone pacemaker implantation for sinoatrial ablation. At age 95 she had dyspnea with minimal exertion. She could no longer walk. An open procedure was too risky. She developed shortness of breath aggravated by physical activity and could only walk 20 feet. She gave consent to having TAVI and three weeks later had only mild shortness of breath on exertion and could walk 10 to 15 feet at a time and walk to a cafeteria. This did not alter the course of the aortic stenosis. Thus here is a procedure that while it does not add years to your life if candidates are carefully selected it can dramatically improve the patients life. The alternative access to using the femoral access that has been described still remains to be proven and accepted. Some patients have too much disease in the femoral artery to permit the femoral approach. A new study will test an alternative approach for TAVR including the apex of the heart, the aorta and the transaxillary and tans subclavian arteries. An estimated 1 in 4 patients are in-eligible because of advanced disease at the approved access site. New clinical guideline will be developed to make recommendations in 26 areas including mechanical valves and biological valves.

In the realm of thoracic surgery and especially cardiac surgery no new procedure has created as large a stir in surgical and world news as cardiac transplantation. This includes cardiac and cardiopulmonary homotransplants. (from other human beings). There is a long history of interest in cardiac transplantation dating back to Carrel and Guthrie when they reported the first cardiac transplant when they reported a cervical heterotopic canine cardiac transplant. There was no further work after about 30 years on the rejection problem until Demikoff who placed the heart in the intrathoracic position. Gibbons work in developing the heart-lung machine in 1953 transformed the whole field and made orthotopic canine transplantation a possibility. In 1960 Lower and Shumway published their landmark work reporting successful canine orthotopic cardiac transplants. It was found that electrocardiograph findings could be used for monitoring rejection by the loss of QRS voltage and arrhythmias. The methods for treating rejection were derived from experience with immunosuppressive agents used in malignancy treatments and experience in the field of renal transplantation. In 1964 the first human transplant was performed by Hardy when they first performed transplantation of a chimpanzee heart into a human, the patient dying in cardiogenic shock. The first successful human was performed by Barnard on Dec, 1967. The patient died of pulmonary infection less than 3 weeks postoperatively, but it generated world- wide interest and enthusiasm. More than 100 cardiac transplants were performed in 1968 but the results were dismal. By 1970 fewer than 20 transplants were done. And the majority of these were done at the Stanford University Medical Center. There has been an improvement both in the numbers and quality since those early days and more than 350 human cardiac transplants performed at Stanford since those early days. And these factors have to do with selection of patients as well as well as the development of a number of very effective immunosuppressive agents such as cyclosporine. Techniques for procuring donors from distant sites enlarge the donor pool greatly and the management of rejection as well as well as a better system of procurement and selection of candidates has made cardiac transplantation a daily reality. Appropriate candidates fall into two pools of patients usually less than55 years of age. The patients fall into two large groups of patients, those with end- stage coronary disease and those with cardiomyopathy. There are strict criteria used for the selection of a suitable donor such as the donor should be less than 35 years of age and not have been subject to prolonged resuscitative procedures. The recipient should not be more than 20% larger and be of the same ABO group. Infection and rejection remain the biggest causes of morbidity and mortality. Graft atherosclerosis remains a common problem after transplantation. Approximately half the patients will experience an episode of rejection during the first postoperative month and 80% will experience it after the first 3 months. Another major problem is graft atherosclerosis. These are felt to be immunologic problems. Sometimes retransplantation has been necessary. Lymphoreticular disease and arrhythmias are occasionally seen in the longterm survivers.

An extension of the heart transplant is logically the heart -lung transplant though results are much less satisfactory. Prolonged survival is mainly lmited by pulmonary disease. The main limitations to its application is the pulmonary disease. There should be no radiographic abnormalities and an adequate p02 on 30% oxygen. Obviously this is a much more demanding project technically and the details are not appropriate to this discussion. Immunosuppression is similar to that used for the heart alone. Baldwin and Shumway reported such transplants in their textbook of surgery and 15 of 25 are surviving with favorable lung and heart function.

Up until now we have concentrated on the blockbusters, the highly technical and scientifically advanced. But that is hardly the end of the list. Statistically the most common cause of death has been coronary artery disease, usually the end result of arteriosclerosis of the coronary arteries by stenosis or complete occlusion by clot at the site of a stenosis. It is a very common disease not necessarily fatal but may be the cause of a number of complicating problems that are the source of pain such as angina, myocardial aneurysm, septal defects, and even localized scarring. These complications are usually of the external visible type but may affect the internal structures such as septum or chordae. Be that as it may coronary stenosis or occlusion are the main culprits and are the main culprits in heart attacks. For some reason attacking the problem on the surface came later than all the attention given to the rheumatic valve problems with all the necessary technical as well as chemical developments necessary for open heart operations. A momentous diagnostic episode occurred in 1958 when Mason Sones of the Cleveland clinic working in the pediatric department found that injecting dye into the coronary artery did not kill the patient and showed that coronary was a segmental disease. This led to the development of the coronary bypass operation with a saphenous vein or an internal mammary artery or sometimes by endarterectomy. This became a world wide phenomena performing 1573cases in one year. Low potassium arrest allowed a quiet field and now 2000 such operations are performed worldwide every 24 hours. Rene Favaloro and Donald Effler were the leaders with the bypass operation.

Pediatric cardiac Surgery

Robert Gross in 1938 introduced the surgical treatment of congenital neart disease when he successfully ligated a patent ductus arteriosus. Blalock and Park described experimental procedures for the treatment of coarctation of the aorta by anastomosis of the subclavian artery to the distal aorta. In the following year Gross, Crafoord and Nylin independently described excision of the coarctation and primary anastomosis to the distal aorta the method that is now preferred. In the following year (1945) Gross and colleges used aortic homografts to bridge the gap after excision of the aortic coarctation. Gross and Ware were the first to recognize that anomalies of the aortic arch caused tracheal or esophageal obstruction that was amenable to surgical correction (1946). In the three decades that followed these milestones there were numerous contributions that clarified the pathophysiology, and the diagnostic and therapeutic variations of these defects. Treatment of patent ductus is considered one of the simplest cardiovascular operations and one of the most curative with little risk to the patient. In the typical case the duct connects the main or left pulmonary artery to the lesser or descending curve of the aortic arch. The ductus normally present during fetal life normally closes after birth usually after 2 weeks but some remain open for up to 1 year. In most cases there are no changes though in some with pulmonary hypertension there may be marked intimal hyperplasia of the medium and small arteries along with muscular hypertrophy and organized clots in the pulmonary arteries. Symptoms can vary widely from none to cardiac failure depending on age and the size of the pulmonary shunt. Some children grow normally with no shortness of breath or other limitations of activity and lead normal lives. In many cases if the ductus is large the additional burden on the heart becomes apparent with shortness of breath, loss of energy and fatigue. Subacute bacterial endocarditis at the site of the ductus is less frequent than it was prior to antibiotics. The typical patent ductus appears to be compatible with a long life if uncorrected but Keys and Shapiro (1943) found that those that are alive at 17 with a patent ductus have a shortened life expectancy about ½ that of the normal population. Campbell concluded on the basis of a review of his own experience that by age 45, 42% of patients with a patent ductus arteriosus will have died. The murmur is a characteristic one and allows an accurate diagnosis of the condition in about 95% of the cases. It is a continuous murmur usually rumbling in systole frequently associated with a thrill which can vary with the size of the shunt. The diagnosis can be confirmed and others excluded on the basis of the murmur, ekg, echocardiogram and roentgenogram. If uncertainty remains the diagnosis can be confirmed by catheterization and cineangiography. Operation is almost always indicated. The risk is small and the only deaths were in infants in failure less than 6 months old. An older patient with pulmonary hypertension and reversed flow in the ductus represents a difficult problem and may not tolerate the surgery.

Other conditions that drew early attention from pediatric cardiac surgeons were aortopulmonary windows and coarctation of the aorta. Aortopulmonary window resembles patent ductus arteriosus in its functional and clinical manifestations. Differential diagnosis can be difficult. The typical fistula is anatomically located just above the aortic valve and varies in size from a few millimeters to several centimeters.

In some instances the defect is located immediately adjacent to the coronary arteries and valves and the condition may be indistinguishable externally from a truncus arteriosus in which the aortic and pulmonary valves are part of a single opening. The clinical manifestations of this condition are practically indistinguishable from a large patent ductus. Cardiac enlargement is almost always present along with physical underdevelopment The murmur is a continuous soft systolic one. The pressure in the two vessels may be equal. Increased pulmonary vascularity often with dilatation of the pulmonary artery is similar to that seen in ductus arteriosus. There is both left and right ventricular hypertrophy in the presence of pulmonary hypertension. The operative risk is higher than with patent ductus arteriosus. This is not a common condition and the technical requirements to correct it can vary from a simple division depending on the size and location of the opening to requiring the heart-lung machine for interruption of circulation and direct vision correction. Results usually show a reduction of heart size and a reduction of pulmonary pressure. Whether the pulmonary bed returns to normal is unknown.

Coarctation of the aorta is an important congenital cardiovascular defect, occurs in a significant number of children an and shortens life if untreated. It usually occurs just distal to the left subclavian artery and occasionally is located in the arch of the aorta itself. In rare instances there is more than one coarctation. It is usually classified as preductal or postductal. In the preductal formerly called infantile because of its association with early death, the pulmonary artery communicates through a large ductus with the distal aorta. There may be additional major intracardiac defects most commonly a ventricular septal defect and in some an atrial septal defect and transposition of the great vessels. The coarctation separates the flow of blood from the left ventricle to the head and arms and the flow from the right ventricle and pulmonary artery to the caudal half of the body through the ductus. This type of coarctation often involves the distal aortic arch along with the isthmus and tends to be more elongated or diffuse. Cardiac failure usually occurs, is intractable and results in death unless correction is possible. It is generally discovered in infancy because of the striking disturbance of circulation by the aortic obstruction in addition to the cardiac defect. Diagnosis is made easily because of the discrepancy of upper and lower pressures. A comparison of radial and femoral pulses and pressures will be diagnostic.

Cases have been described in which both subclavian arteries arose from the region of the coarctation and were hypoplastic. Consequently there was no brachial hypertension. In such patients observation of collateral circulation is most important for the diagnosis. In addition to the pathognomonic pulse and pressure gradient, there are often pulsations in the neck and supraclavicular area due to hypertension. There may be diastolic murmurs and systolic murmurs over the base of the heart or in the back. The heart may show some increase in size but when is unduly large other anomalies must be considered. Notching of the ribs is common due to the collateral circulation. The EKG may vary from normal to left ventricular hypertrophy. Coarctation is an important cause of cardiac failure in infants. Most of the deaths in infants with coarctation occur in young ones with preductal coarctation, usually with intracardiac defects. Adults with typical postductal coarctation have an abbreviated life expectancy. Most die before their 40th year. Blalock and Park reported an operation designed to bypass the coarctation by anastomosing the left subclavian artery to the distal aorta. This operation was not attempted until Crafoord and Nylin (1945) and Gross and Hufnagel (1945) did so independently. This became the standard operation. Results found in 1601 patients the average mortality was 8.6%. The mortality was lower in patients between the ages of 4 and 15 years. Among the patients who survived satisfactory relief of hypertension was obtained in 95.2%. And entirely normal readings were found in in 72%. One complication which appears to be an unfortunate byproduct of the relief of hypertension has been necrotizing arteritis and although rare it has occasionally been fatal. A rare and distressing complication has been paraplegia or weakness of the lower part of the body after operation reported by Brewer. In the late 1960s several reports of recurrent coarctation appeared. The ultimate results of treatment of coarctation are unknown. In a study of patients followed for 25 years there was a high incidence of cardiovascular disease, 78% in one special group. Percutaneous transluminal balloon angioplasty has been recommended in selected patients with recurrent stenosis with successful results. In another report percutaneous transluminal angioplasty was successfully used to treat coarctation restenosis and it successfully reduced the systolic gradient across the coactation from a mean of 58 to 13 after the procedure.

Of 160 babies operated on byRobert Gross 40% had a double arch, 25% had a right arch and left ligamentum arteriosum, 12% had an anomalous innominate or carotid artery, 19% had an aberrant right subclavian artery, and 13% had miscellaneous other anomalies. These are really challenging anomalies to correct particularly because there are so many variations. Each is a unique problem that tests not only the surgeons skill but his judgement in picking the right operation.

Atrial and Ventricular Septal Defect

The story of attempts to close atrial and ventricular septal defects is one of attempts to correct these defects using closed techniques that is by passing sutures from outside the heart but before open heart techniques were available followed by the magic of hypothermia with its limited time inside the heart and finally the heart-lung machine that allowed direct vision surgery especially important for the more complicated lesions. Gordon Murray of Canada in 1948 reported on his experiments in dogs first and then operated on 4 patients. He passed sutures from a point just distal to the annulus fibrosis and slightly to the right of the descending branch of the left coronary artery. and then out between the superior venacava and the pulmonary veins. All of his patients recovered but nothing was said of the results. In 1950 Sondergaard described his technique for the closure of atrial septal defects and in 1954 reported his experience in3 patients. Crafoord suggested placing a finger in the atrium while placing the blind sutures but there were recurrences. In 1952 Bailey reported his treatment of atrial septal defects called atrioseptopexy and put his finger into the atrium to guide his sutures. Since using his technique he operated on five patients with two deaths.

In 1952 Lewis and associates at the University of Minnesota successfully closed an atrial defect under hypothermia. After this the technique was used throughout the world. In 1953 Gross introduced the atrial well made of rubber which he sewed to the atrial wall. The blood pressure in the atrium was so low that the blood did not escape from the atrium. He operated on 7 patients with this technique with good results. He eventually gave up this technique because he felt that serious regurgitation was aggravated. He continued the use of a closed technique for septal defects with practically no mortality. Bailey in 1955 said that since 1952 he had operated on 73 patients using the so-called atrioseptopexy technique. There had been 57 secundum defects (atrial) with 5deaths. There had been 16 primum defects and he had lost 60% of these. The first patient to be operated upon successfully for closure of an atrial septal defect using an extracorporeal pump-oxygenator was done by Gibbon on May 6, 1953. This was the first time that an oxygenator had been successfully used to allow for a direct open operation on the heart with blood diverted to the pump-oxygenator and returned to the patient usually by a cannula in the femoral artery or the aorta. She was connected to the apparatus for 45 minutes and for 26 minutes all cardiorespiratory function was taken over by the machine. The defect was closed easily with a continuous silk suture and the patient made an uneventful recovery. Actually the very first closures of ventricular septal defects was by Lillehei using a controlled cross circulation from parent to child in 1954. Development of the pump-oxygenator in 1953 eventually supplanted all other techniques.

Kay, Kirklin and Lillehei all made early contributions to the techniques of closure of ventricular septal defects and even the more complicated tetralogy of Fallot. One of the extreme problems of ventricular septal defect is the complete absence of a septum. Maude Abbott found in 1000 autopsies on patients with congenital heart disease two hundred and seventy four ventricular septal defects and three hundred and seventy three atrial defects. The venricular defect may be in the anterior or posterior part of the septum. Associated with these defects may be abnormal positions of the aortic and pulmonary trunks. Many of the defects lie below or in the outflow tracts. There may be multiple defects. The conduction system lies close to the posterior inferior margin of the defect and care must be taken not to pass sutures through it. In the operation the large quantity of blood makes the closure difficult. Because sutures cut through the delicate tissue an Ivalon patch is usually used. The use of temporary extracorporeal bypass in the surgical treatment of cardiac and aortic diseases was described by Cooley, Debakey and associates in 1957. They withdrew blood from the venae cavae and returned it to the femoral artery instead of the subclavian as was done at first. They used a modification of the

DeWall-Lillehei oxygenator with special stainless steel oxygen diffuser. Dow Coming antifoam as well as a polyethylene bottle were used to debubble the blood after it came from the oxygenator. They used an incision carried across the sternum rather than the sternal splitting approach that most surgeons used. Closure of ventricular septal defects in 45 cases was attended with seven deaths (27%). In 1957 Lillehei and associates reported on their experience with open-heart surgery for congenital heart disease. They had used three types of extracorporeal circulation at the University of Minnesota in the last two years and finally came to using a a disposable plastic bubble diffusion oxygenator. One hundred and fifty-four patients with ventricular septal defects had been operated upon. The lethal element of ventricular septal defect is the early rapid and progressive development of pulmonary hypertension associated with a high pulmonary vascular resistance. The initiating and determining factor is the systolic thrust of the left ventricular output delivered undamped to the pulmonary vessels. There were forty-five deaths with an overall mortality of 29.3%.

CHAPTER 3

Hypothermia

HYPOTHERMIA WITH INDUCED cardiac arrest is the other aspect of the use of hypothermia in cardiac surgery. In 1955 Melrose (England) described elective cardiac arrest as an adjunct to operations on the open heart. Hooker's work in 1929 was the basis for much of the techniques used later to produce cardiac arrest by injection of potassium chloride into the coronaries which would result in a flaccid heart for the surgeon to operate on. Restoration could be accomplished by a variety of maneuvers such as injection of a solution of calcium chloride, or cardiac massage, sometimes adrenalin or neostigmine or just restoration of circulation. Restoration of muscle tone was always followed by fibrillation usually requiring electrical defibrillation. With the use of the heart-lung machine the aortic clamp is released followed by perfusion of the coronary arteries which restores tone and normal rhythm without the need for other drugs. It should be noted that many operators at some point in developing their techniques would perfuse the coronary arteries while working on the aortic valve with the reasoning that cold oxygenated blood was the best way to protect the myocardium while doing the procedure. As usual some devised cocktails of oxygenated blood and drugs to protect the heart while the surgeon operated on the valve. It was also common to protect the heart using straight hypothermia such as iced saline poured over the heart before opening the heart and sometimes leaving the heart sit in cold saline while working on the valve. Obviously much attention was given to preserving good myocardial function even to the point of developing new defibrillators such as the direct current defibrillator by Bernard

Lown MD a Boston Cardiologist. If all this activity in the 1950s doesn't impress you there is more.

With all this activity operating on diseased valves of the heart was very difficult because of the technical difficulties of producing adequate hypothermia, cardiac arrest, limited operating time and the possible damage to other organs. In 1953 John H Gibbon used an extracorporeal 'Heart-Lung Machine' developed with the aid of IBM to give the patient continuous blood flow during an open heart procedure. Credit must be given also to the contributions of Clarence Dennis who in 1951 performed the first known open cardiotomy with mechanical takeover of the heart and lungs at the University of Minnesota Hospital however the patient did not survive the operation. In 1951 Dr William T Mustard also developed a heart-lung machine but little is known of its original application. Charles Best produced heparin about this same time essential to prevent clotting of blood which was a significant danger when so much blood is exposed to so many foreign surfaces. Dr John Gibbon is credited with the first open heart operation during a 26 minute extrcorporeal bypass on May 6, 1953 closing a large atrial septal defect. This changed the world of heart surgery. The construction and design of the heart-lung machine was destined to undergo many changes with time. This would involve the design, synthetic materials in the oxygenator, and the ability to produce total body hypothermia.

The success treating mitral stenosis with a closed technique could not be repeated with aortic valve stenosis also a common complication of rheumatic heart disease. Of the valvular diseases complicating rheumatic fever this was the next most common and just as incapacitating. Leonardo Da Vinci illustrated the aortic valve as the exit from the heart with three cusps two situated posteriorly and one anteriorly at the base of the aorta. The free margins of each cusp are thickened and strengthened by tendinous fibers that form the corpora aranti. Pulse duplicator studies reveal that the cusps press against each other and support each other in closure at the end of a ventricular contraction. The coronary artery orifices are located above two of the cusps. Thus this small bit of anatomy plays an important role not just for circulation of blood to the body but also is crucial to the circulation of the heart. Parts of the posterior and left cusps are continuous with the major leaflet of the mitral valve thus making this valve susceptible to damage if there is aneurysmal dilatation or dissection at the base of the aorta. Aortic stenosis (narrowing of the opening restricting blood flow) may be of congenital, rheumatic, or arteriosclerotic origin. It may be calcific (bony hard) or non- calcific. The congenital aortic stenosis may be isolated or it may associated with coarctation of the aorta (narrowing) or it may be bicuspid (two leaflets instead of three) with an eccentric orifice the kind commonly found when operated on later in life. It is often difficult to determine whether a heavily calcified valve was originally bicuspid or tricuspid. Rheumatic fever is the most common cause of aortic stenosis in the adult. The progressive fibrosis and calcification may produce valves that are completely immobile with no semblance of normal anatomic markings. Calcific deposits may produce a valve that is more than a centimeter thick and may involve the atrioventricular node, the bundle of His, the coronary ostia or the mitral valve. Concomitant involvement of the mitral and tricuspid valves is not unusual. The entire valve and adjacent structures may be completely replaced by calcium. Extension of calcification to the bundle of His in the membranous septum may result in complete atrioventricular dissociation and chronic heart block. These are serious rhythm problems of the heart especially the extremely slow heart rate of heart block. Secondary changes in the size and weight of the left ventricle (hypertrophy) as well as changes in the thickness of the right ventricle are not unusual with tight aortic valve stenosis.

The pathology of the valve as well as the anatomy at the base of the aorta made a closed approach (not direct vision) difficult. These account for the more reluctant approach surgically to correcting aortic stenosis and certainly absence of a closed approach for correction of aortic insufficiency (leakage backwards at the valve). The attempts at correcting aortic stenosis consisted of sewing a tube onto the wall of the aorta for the insertion of a finger or an instrument since there was no appendage like there was at the left or right atrium and the so-called transventricular approach or inserting an instrument through the apex of the left ventricle that could be used to dilate the aortic orifice or a knife to incise the valve hopefully at the commisures. Surgically no approach was attempted to correct aortic stenosis until Tuffier in 1912 operated upon a patient with a thrill over the aorta. He pushed in the aortic wall under the ring penetrating far into the area of the stenosis and the thrill became less marked. The patient recovered from the operation and returned home. In 1950 Bailey operated using the transventricular knife and she died. Intolerable regurgitation was felt to be the problem. In April 1950 he operated on a patient by passing an instrument with an umbrella like dilator down the common carotid artery. She recovered. Twice again he did this operation and one died. He then shifted to the transventricular approach and between 1950 and 1952 he did 11 operations. A new dilator was perfected and he then carried out many operations. In 1956 he and associates reported on two hundred and eighty-seven patients using the transventricular approach. In April 1953 Bailey carried out a transaortic operation on the aortic valve. He made a pouch of pericardium and sutured it to the aorta so that he could insert his finger or instrument through it without loss of blood. Of 68 patients followed one to three years after a transventricular operation there had been an operative mortality of 28%. Eighty-five percent were improved. Forty-seven had been operated on by the transaortic route with an operative mortality of 14%. These were astounding results for a difficult and inpenetrable as well as disabling lesion of the aortic valve. In 1958 Glover reported a followup study of 50 patients who had commisurotomy four and one half to seven years previously. About three-fourths were in better condition and leading more normal lives. In 1957 Bailey discussed recurrent mitral stenosis.

Up until now there has not been a creditable operation for mitral or aortic insufficiency (incompetence of the valve or backward flow through the valve after a contraction of the ventricle). The next step on the road to direct vision correction of the malfunction or destruction of the valve by disease or by congenital malformation was to find a way to stop circulation through the valve without interfering with the blood flow to the body or to reduce the need for oxygen and blood flow by reducing the metabolism to a point that allowed stopping circulation for a short period of time. The history of the application of hypothermia to allow interruption of blood flow to the heart or even blood flow to the body is clouded by a variety of techniques and limited successes over the span of time though mostly in the 1950s. We need to separate the efforts to reduce total body temperature for the purposes of interrupting circulation to the whole body for a short time and interrupting circulation to the heart while working on the valve. Both of these were technical problems that were worked on in the dog laboratory in the 40s and applied successfully in the 50s. The contribution of Bigelow and his many associates in the dog lab was followed by a successful open heart operation in dogs using hypothermia in 1950 followed by a successful human case in 1954 at the Toronto General Hospital. The total body temperature was lowered and the blood entering the heart was stopped and the heart was opened for 20 minutes. Hypothermia became the most common form of open-heart surgery till about 1960. The first successful open-heart operation using the heart-lung machine was carried out by John Gibbon in 1953 and this was combined with hypothermia about 1960.

Hypothermia with induced cardiac arrest is the other aspect of the use of hypothermia in cardiac surgery. In 1955 Melrose (England) described elective cardiac arrest as an adjunct to operations on the open heart. Hooker's work in 1929 was the basis for much of the techniques used later to produce cardiac arrest by injection of potassium chloride into the coronaries which would result in a flaccid heart for the surgeon to operate on. Restoration could be accomplished by a variety of maneuvers such as injection of a solution of calcium chloride, or cardiac massage, sometimes adrenalin or neostigmine or just restoration of circulation. Restoration of muscle tone was always followed by fibrillation usually requiring electrical defibrillation. With the use of the heart-lung machine the aortic clamp is released followed by perfusion of the coronary arteries which restores tone and normal rhythm without the need for other drugs. It should be noted that many operators at some point in developing their techniques would perfuse the coronary arteries while working on the aortic valve with the reasoning that cold oxygenated blood was the best way to protect the myocardium while doing the procedure. As usual some devised cocktails of oxygenated blood and drugs to protect the heart while the surgeon operated on the valve. It was also common to protect the heart using straight hypothermia such as iced saline poured over the heart before opening the heart and sometimes leaving the heart sit in cold saline while working on the valve. Obviously much attention was given to preserving good myocardial function even to the point of developing new defibrillators such as the direct current defibrillator by Bernard Lown MD a Boston Cardiologist. If all this activity in the 1950s doesn't impress you there is more.

With all this activity operating on diseased valves of the heart was very difficult because of the technical difficulties of producing adequate hypothermia, cardiac arrest, limited operating time and the possible damage to other organs. In 1953 John H Gibbon used an extracorporeal 'Heart-Lung Machine' developed with the aid of IBM to give the patient continuous blood flow during an open heart procedure. Credit must be given also to the contrbutions of Clarence Dennis who in 1951 who performed the first known open cardiotomy with mechanical takeover of the heart and lungs at the University of Minnesota Hospital however the patient did not survive the operation. In 1951 Dr William T Mustard also developed a heart-lung machine but little is known of its original application. Charles Best produced heparin about this same time essential to prevent clotting of blood which was a significant danger when so much blood is exposed to so many foreign surfaces. Dr John Gibbon is credited with the first open heart operation during a 26 minute extrcorporeal bypass on May 6, 1953 closing a large atrial septal defect. This changed the world of heart surgery. The construction and design of the heart-lung machine was destined to undergo many changes with time. This would involve the design and synthetic materials in the oxygenator, the ability to produce total body hypothermia, filters for the blood to remove platelet aggregation, the addition of pumps for suction of blood from the operative field and a variety of priming solutions from straight unadulterated blood to bloodless ionic solutions. The original oxygenator which was large and cumbersome was soon replaced by the bubble oxygenator developed by De Wall and Lillehei at the University of Minnesota. While this gained wide acceptance there were soon problems evident in the blood and patient related to the blood-gas interphase and this was later supplanted by a membrane oxygenator. The development of the current membrane oxygenator is also the result of many laboratory experiments and basically composed as a tube of blood which contains many small tubes of permeable silastic through which a mixture of oxygen-carbon dioxide flows so that there is no blood- gas interphase.

The history of the oxygenator dates back to 1885 with the first demonstration of a disc oxygenator. on which blood was exposed to the atmosphere on rotating discs by Von Frey and Gruber. They noted the dangers of blood streaming, foaming and clotting. Working independently, Brukonenko in the USSR and John Heysham Gibbon in the USA demonstrated the feasability of extracorporeal oxygenation. Brukonenko used excised dog lungs while Gibbon used a direct contact drum type oxygenator, perfusing cats for up to 25 minutes in the 1930s.

Gibbons first successful operation on a human used a stationary film type in which oxygen was exposed to a film of blood as it flowed over a series of stainless steel plates. The first membrane artificial lung was demonstrated in 1955 by a group led by Willem Kolff and in 1956 the first disposable membrane oxygenator removed the need for time consuming cleaning before reuse. The highly permeable silicone rubber membranes were introduced in the 1960s and as hollow fibers in 1971 which revollutionized the design of membrane disposable modules.

Operations which involve uncoated cardiopulmonary bypass circuits require a high dose of systemic heparin. Although heparin is reversible by administering protamine there are side effects whch can include allergic reaction resulting in thrombocytopenia and various reactions to the administration of protamine as well as post-operative hemorrhage due to inadequate reversal of the anticoagulant. Systemic heparin does not completely prevent clotting or the activation of complement, neutrphils and monocytes which are the principal mediators of the inflammatory response. This response produces a wide range of cytotoxins and cell-signalling proteins that circulate throughout he patients body during surgery and disrupt homeostasis. This inflammatory response can produce problems in the patient during bypass and in the postoperative period. Other problems may stem from a certain amount of surgical debris and lipids. Micoparticles can obstruct arterioles that supply small nests of cells throughout the body and together with cytotoxins damage organs and tissue and temporarily disturb organ function. All aspects of cardiopulmonary bypass, including manipulation of the aorta may be associated with neurological symptoms following bypass. Such temporary neuological symptoms are sometimes referred to as "pumphead syndrome". Heparin-coated blood oxygenators are one option to decrease morbidity associated with cardio-pulmonary bypass but the advantages appear very limited. Brain injury appears to be a significant though temporary problem in patients undergoing cardiac surgery assisted by cardiopulmonary bypass due to numerous acellular lipid deposits (10-70um) in the micro-vasculature due to cadiotomy suction presumably because of lipid microembolization. Impaired kidney function is ocasionally noted as a result of prolonged bypass.

But we are now at the stage in our development that allows us to review an array of corrective operations that were suddenly possible after the mid 50s revolution. Who would have thought after the first closed correction of mitral stenosis using the blind finger in the atrial appendage that we would soon be able to correct the diseased valves under direct vision, remove and replace valves using a variety of ball valves or homograft valves or treated animal valves, or disc valves or remove tumours of the heart, or close defects with woven plastic materials, pace the heart when needed with sophistiated pacemaker-defibrillators, replace the aorta with new woven materials, and finally replace the whole heart or lung or heart and lungs as a unit with controlled rejection. In addition there are now an array of pumps and artificial hearts that can be used on a temporary basis until a suitable transplant is available. All of these are a tribute to the ingenuity, the laboratory research, and the drive of the surgeons and the industrial counterparts who cooperated with the surgeons and the laboratories to bring this about. The Institutes of Health played major supporting rolls by supporting grants.

En Passant we should mention the singular events that led us to the sophistication that we now enjoy, the possibilities of the advanced cardiopulmonary bypass that we now enjoy. In the early 50s hypothermia was the sole method for open-heart surgery but its survival was short because it was cumbersome, difficult to achieve the safe levels of total body hypothermia, usually by the use of blankets through which was circulated ice cold water until temperatures as measured by a rectal thermometer reached 30 degrees centigrade. There were attempts at surface cooling in a bath tub filled with ice water and the surgeon was limited to straightforward operations because of the speed and skill needed for a 6 to 10 minute operating time. Cooling continues to be a part of modern bypass systems in the form of heat exchangers but is no longer a limiting factor on time. The names of surgeons associated with the development of hypothermia in open heart surgery are Wilfred Cordon Bigelow in Canada, John Lewis in Minneapolis, and Henry Swan the leader in the field at the University of Colorado.

Henry Swan carried out his first open-heart procedure using hypothermia at the University of Colorado on February 19,1953. He excised a stenosed pulmonic valve during a 7 1/2 min inflow occlusion. Swan went on to become the surgeon with the greatest experience with hypothermia in hundreds of cases with a very low mortality. Bigelow and Swan will always be associated with hypothermia in cardiac surgery.

Charles Drew and Price Thomas perfomed many operations at the Brompton and Westminster Hospitals London in the 1960s.

Another fundamental contribution of that same era is the development of the cardiac pacemaker. Bigelow and co-workers reported on a still clumsy pacemaker in 1950 but Paul Zoll, a Boston cardiologist reported the first successful clinical use of a pacemaker in 1952. Lillehei in 1957 used a wire electrode sutured to the myocardium bringing it out to an external machine. Ake Senning is credited with the first implantable pacemaker in 1958.

The advent of the Heart-Lung machine changed the world of heart surgery. Although the cross circulation technique of Lillehei and the adventures of Bigelow, Swann and Lewis in closing ventricular and septal defects and perhaps closing an associated valve defect the operating time inside the heart was too limited for the more complex and . . . time consuming operations on all the valves of the adult as well as the pediatric heart. Some aortic and mitral stenotic valves were so destroyed and calcified by disease that that they required replacement though there were those, particularly mitral insufficiency and aortic insufficiency that lent themselves to reconstruction or tightening the annulus. This was particularly true for tricuspid valve insufficiency which was not very common.

The story of total valve replacement dates to the late 1950s when Mueller reconstructed a resected aortic valve using a trcuspid prosthesis made of Teflon cloth in December 1958. In 1960 Harken implanted the first sub-coronary ball valve. Roe et al used a molded tricuspid silastic valve in the subcoronary area. The ball valve was accepted as the standard for aortic valve prosthetic replacement. The Starr-Edwards aortic ball valves were sold from 1962 to 1965 and more than 10,000 valves of steel, titanium and stellite construction were sold. The first subcoronary ball valve placed in March 1960, had to be replaced after 31 /2 years because of parabasilar leakage. Review of 860 balls returned to Edwards for examination and evaluation did reveal some signs of loss of volume and injury and biodegradation followed by death but the later series (1200 to 1260) appeared almost free of the problem. One problem that accompanied all the prosthetics of the caged varieties was the tendecy to develop thrombus on the cage and even embolization which led to design modificatons and long-term anticoagulation. Design changes for the metal parts of the valve included cloth covered struts and a hollow titanium metal ball. Despite these changes surgeons began to swing their preferences to discoid valves. In 1963 Ross reported his early results with subcoronary homograft aortic valve transplants using freeze-dried formalin fixed and frozen grafts. Barret-Boyes subsequently reported an extensive and very successful experience with freeze-dried homograft aortic valve replacement in aortic stenosis and aortic insufficiency. The next trend was the use of frame mounted heterologous (animal source) valves and the tilting disc valve as described by Bjork later by Lillehei. The techniques to preserve the myocardium were used almost universally and these included coronary perfusion with cold blood, bathing the heart in iced saline and perfusion with cold ionic solutions containing not only sugar and sodium chloride but other chemicals that might be of research interest. No need to go into the many technical details of sutures, body temperature, heparin anticoagulation, blood flows, carbon dioxide levels and oxygen levels as well blood transfusions. Suffice it to say that restoration of normal coronary perfusion after the aorta or the heart is closed is usually accompanied by good coarse fibrillation of the heart and an easy defibrillation to normal sinus rythm.

The story of treating mitral Insufficiency varies widely from that of mitral senosis because it really required direct vision of the valve and in most cases an artificial valve rather than a reconstruction though both approaches had their followers and quite successfully. We will first discuss the ball valve approach since it came first in the long series of valves that have been tried and used in the rather fierce competition of designers and manufacturers for the market. The early experimenters in the early years, and there were many in the first part of the twentieth century, tried vein slings as well as circumferential sutures around the annulus of the heart were attended by occasional success but the mortality rate was more than could be tolerated. Some names that might be mentioned are Murray (1938), Bailey (1955), and Glover in 1955 with the circumferential suture around the annulus. Scott and associates in 1957 reported their experiernce in the surgical correction of mitral isufficiency under direct vision. Two recovered and 2 died. Effler of Cleveland at the 1958 Meeting reported that he had operated on 14 patients and had used cardiac arrest in all of them. He believed that the ultimate operation for the condition would be the use of a plastic valve. There didn't seem to be a preference as to which side of the chest was preferred in their surgical approach, many more used the right side. Effler had operated on 16 patients wth mitral insufficiency and lost four of them. The pathology of the valve can vary widely. Somtimes the commissures are fused and easily separated at other tmes there is subvalvular fusion and calcification that cannot be easily separated or reconstructed. In such cases valve replacemt is the obvious and only answer. The degree of heart enlargement due to the mammoth size of the left atrium in those wth free regurge at the mitral valve is truly impressive.

Occasionally a mitral valve can be repaired or 'fixed' but this is not common and an artificial valve must be chosen for replacement. These now come in various designs. The prosthetic valve first reported by Starr and Edwards in 1961 is very similar and amost identical to the Harken aortic valve and were introduced at about the same time. Minor variations were introduced with time but both had a teflon sewing ring, a metal 4 domed cage of stainless steel or titanium and usually a hollow silastc ball. These worked well in the dynamics required of an aortic and /mitral valve. The silastic ball valves of Starr and Harken were folllowed by modifications that led through a variety of low-profile disc valves, cloth-covered valves and mounted homograft valves and heterograft valves. The surgeon's choice is determined by his experience both with thrombosis and durability. The annuloplasty technique of Carpentier et al using a cloth covered steel ring has merit. There are three operative approaches to the mitral valve and each requires minor modifications of the pumping technique, The sternal splitting incision is the most versatile because it allows access to all chambers of the heart and to the aorta with the least postoperative interference with pulmonary function. Chronic mitral insufficiecy associated with a giant left atrium usually can be handled with a right or left thoracotomy. These are technical details that the surgeon must come to grips with when planning an operation. Cannulation of the superior and inferior vena cava is performed in the standard fashion and the common femoral artery or the ascending aorta are cannulated for arterial return. Cold potssium cardioplegia induced, the apex of the left ventricle is elevated and a catheter introduced for suction while the valve is sewn in place using multiple sutures at the annulus. As the wall of the left atrium is closed all air in the left ventricle and atrium is removed through the previously placed catheter and the heart allowed to resume function using a defibrillator if need be.

In evaluating results it is important to separate realistic current statistics from from those in the development stage. Patients in a class III category, will do better on the improvement and mortality scales as time goes on and the surgeon gains experience in selecting patients and best valve. Some examples. For example Kittle et al reported on 216 patients using the the Starr-Edwards valve wth a hospital mortality for the ball valve of 23%. Litwak et al reported 110 patients with mortality of 12.7%. Reis et al reported a hospital mortality of 8%. Such are the vagaries of mortality figures and the important vagaries of patient selection, unforseen or unexplained complications and the effects that so many variables can have. Complications with the brain or the kidneys, or even blood interaction with foreign material can have unexpected consequences such as stroke or kidney failure. These are not all failures, or deaths but they do illustrate possible and worrisome problems, many of which will clear or improve with treatment and time. Hospital Mortality early in the reporting results varied from 2% to 32% and the late mortality varied from 2% to 39%. These are not the only valve problems that show up on the schedule. Pulmonic valve stenosis as well aortic stenosis are part of the congenital spectrum of valve problems and was one of the earliest open hearts done under hypothermic arrest. We should mention mutivalvular disease as part our discussion simply because it is not common but because in advanced cases of heart disease involving two or three of the major valves of the heart of the adult patient threre may be a need to replace the aortic, the mitral and less often the tricuspid valves at the same operation. Obviously it can be done at the same operation but requires stamina on the part of the surgeon as well as meticulous preparation on the part of the whole team. Two valves at the same operation is a trial of your expertise and management. Three magnifies the strain on the whole team as well as the prolonged time on the pump-oxygenator and the possible complications. The results of such blockbuster operations are not as spectacular as those that involve one valve or even two valves but short of a total heart replacement. Correction of one lesion without appreciation of the associated hemodynamically significant lesion has led to death during the procedure or immediately after. Combined valvular disease is present in 12 to 30% of patients with aortic or mitral stenosis. The clinical features of combined aortic and mitral disease are dominated by the mitral disease.

Operations which involve uncoated(Cardio-pulmonary bypass) circuits require a high dose of systemic heparin. Although the effects of heparin are reversible by administering protamine, there are a number of side effects associated with this. Side effects can include allergic reaction to heparin resulting in thrombocytopenia, various reactions to the administration of protamine and post-operative hemorrhage due to inadequate reversal of the anticoagulation. Systemic heparin does not completely prevent clotting or the activation of complement, neutrophils, and monocytes, which are the principal mediators of the inflammatory response. This response produces a wide range of cytotoxins, and cell-signaling proteins that circulate throughout the patient's body during surgery and disrupt homeostasis. The inflammatory responses can produce microembolic particles. A greater source of such microemboli are caused by the suction of surgical debris and lipids into the CPB circuit.[1]

Microparticles obstruct arterioles that supply small nests of cells throughout the body and, together with cytotoxins, damage organs and tissues and temporarily disturb organ function. All aspects of cardiopulmonary bypass, including manipulation of the aorta by the surgeon, may be associated with neurological symptoms following perfusion. Physicians refer to such temporary neurological deficits as "pumphead syndrome." Heparin-coated blood oxygenators are one option available to a surgeon and a perfusionist to decrease morbidity associated with CPB to a limited degree.

Heparin-coated oxygenators are thought to:

- Improve overall biocompatibility and host homeostasis
- Mimic the natural endothelial lining of the vasculature
- Reduce the need for systemic anticoagulation
- Better maintain platelet count
- Reduce adhesion of plasma proteins
- Prevent denaturation and activation of adhered proteins and blood cells
- Avoid complications resulting from an abnormal pressure gradient across the oxygenator

Surgical outcomes

Heparin coating is reported to result in similar characteristics to the native endothelium. It has been shown to inhibit intrinsic coagulation, inhibit host responses to extracorporeal circulation, and lessen postperfusion, or "pumphead," syndrome. Several studies have examined the clinical efficacy of these oxygenators.

Up until now there has not been a creditable operation for mitral or aortic insufficiency (incompetence of the valve or backward flow through the valve after a contraction of the ventricle). The next step on the road to direct vision correction of the malfunction or destruction of the valve by disease or by congenital malformation was to find a way to stop circulation through the valve without interfering with the blood flow to the body or to reduce the need for oxygen and blood flow by reducing the metabolism to a point that allowed stopping circulation for a short period of time. The history of the application of hypothermia to allow interruption of blood flow to the heart or even blood flow to the body is clouded by a variety of techniques and limited successes over the span of time though mostly in the 1950s. We need to separate the efforts to reduce total body temperature for the purposes of interrupting circulation to the whole body for a short time and interrupting circulation to the heart while working on the valve. Both of these were technical problems that were worked on in the dog laboratory in the 40s and applied successfully in the 50s. The contribution of Bigelow and his many associates in the dog lab was followed by a successful open heart operation in dogs using hypothermia in 1950 followed by a successful human case in 1954 at the Toronto General Hospital. The total body temperature was lowered and the blood entering the heart was stopped and the heart was opened for 20 minutes. Hypothermia became the most common form of open-heart surgery till about 1960. The first successful open-heart operation using the heart-lung machine was carried out by John Gibbon in 1953 and this was combined with hypothermia about 1960.

CHAPTER 4

The Heart-Lung Machine

THE HEART-LUNG MACHINE has made most of the advances possible that occurred during the past century. Like all advances there is a preliminary history of pioneers and developmental steps. Like its name the heart-lung machine is composed of an oxygenator for oxygenating venous blood and one or more pumps for returning blood to the patient to provide circulation. The oxygenator has a longer history than the pumps that are currently in use.

The history of the oxygenator dates back to 1885 with the first demonstration of a disc oxygenator in which blood was exposed to an atmosphere of oxygen on rotating discs by Frey and Gruber. They noted the dangers of blood streaming, foaming and clotting. Working independently, Brukonenko in the USSR and John Heysham Gibbon in the USA demonstrated the feasibility of extracorporeal oxygenation. Again the 1950s was the setting for significant advances and three men made it all possible Gibbon, Kirklin and Lillehei.

John Gibbon will be remembered as the man who, after 22 years of persistent research developed the first successful heart-lung machine. Gibbon used a direct contact drum type oxygenator perfusing cats for up to 25 minutes in the 1930s. Gibbons first successful operation on a human in 1953 used a stationary film type in which oxygen was exposed to a film of blood as it flowed over a series of stainless steel plates. The first membrane artificial lung was demonstrated in 1955 by a group led by a Willem Kolff and in 1956 the first disposable membrane oxygenator removed the need for time consuming cleaning before reuse. The highly gas permeable silicone rubber membranes were introduced in the 1960s and as hollow fibers in 1971 which revolutionized the design of membrane disposable nodules. Gibbons background is interesting in that he was a research fellow with Churchill, then went to Philadelphia to practice surgery, obtained another research fellowship with Churchill then in 1946 met Thomas Watson, the Chairman of IBM who agreed to support the project financially and give technical assistance. This association apparently provided the needed breakthrough. In 1951 John and Mary Gibbon was able to report on seven dogs surviving and on May 6, 1953 he performed the first open heart operation using extracorporeal circulation. His patient, Cecelia Bavolek, had a large atrial septal defect repaired during a 26 minute cardio-pulmonary bypass. Following this epochal success Gibbon lost the next four patients and abandoned all further attempts, an attitude that puzzled many experts and was even criticized by some. It may be that at the age of 50 he had lost the drive to wrestle with the problems of open-heart surgery. John Kirklin obtained Gibbon's authorization and had the machine perfected with the help of the MAYO physiology and engineering departments. John Kirklin was an exceptional technical surgeon and a far seeing investigator as was Lillehei. Both had their share of firsts and we shall hear more about Lillehi further on. They both belonged to that special Minneapolis and Minnesota group that ruled the world of heart surgery in their day.

Simultaneously Forsmann, Cournand, and Richards developed cardiac catheterization that permitted anatomical and physiological diagnosis of heart disease during life. And about the same time there was the discovery and commercial production of heparin that was necessary for the use of the heart-lung. This anticoagulant was essential for the use of the heart-lung machine because of the extensive foreign surfaces in a heart-lung machine. Without this anticoagulant passage of blood through the pump-oxygenator would be complicated by clotting that would cause serious damage to all organs and death of the patient. It is fortunate that these developments were in place at the time Gibbons was ready with his contribution. We need to remember that the machine we call a pump-oxygenator consists of long lines of polyethylene tubing that drains the venous blood to the oxygenator through a compression pump and reservoir and back to the patient again from the oxygenator and a reservoir through a long length of polyethylene tubing and another compression pump. Blood in the body does not clot because the entire system is lined by endothelial cells that are clot resistant. But even with a full dose of heparin and continuous checks of the clotting time and a full dose of heparin some tolerable changes occur in the blood and these can include allergic reactions resulting in thrombocytopenia, reactions to the protamine given to reverse the heparin. Systemic heparin does not completely prevent clotting or the activation of complement, neutrophils, and monocytes which are the principal mediators of the inflammatory response. This response produces a wide range of cytotoxins, and cell signaling proteins. There are complications to look for because of these changes as well as changes in the blood from suctioning blood from the operative field. Certain organs such as the kidneys and even the brain may show signs of damage temporarily and occasionally of a serious and permanent nature. Thrombocytopenia and bleeding are signs to look for immediately postop because much of this can be corrected by a transfusion of thrombocytes.

Walt Lillehei is certainly one of the most interesting characters in the realm of cardiac surgery. He is best known for the early use of cross circulation and the bubble oxygenator. Both were milestones in the development of open heart surgery. He was one of that remarkable group under Owen Wangesteen at the University of Minnesota in the 1950s that did so much to advance the concepts and use of open-heart surgery.

On the road to open-heart surgery he became interested in a paper on low-flow physiology by Anthony Andreasen in the 1952 British Journal of Surgery. He looked into the the practical possibilities of low flow circulation for extracorporeal circulation. They named the phenomenon that an animal's brain survived with only a small fraction of the total blood volume the 'azygos flow principle'. Lillehei's background in the North African Campaign and his fight with parotid malignancy and radical head, neck and mediastinal surgery undoubtedly shaped his world. When he presented his ideas about cross circulation between a patient and a human donor, Clarence Dennis (Lillehei's senior) thought that "I was some kind of nut" and when he later presented his clinical series of cross-circulation Willis Potts, a noted cardiac surgeon ironically suggested that the author had just presented an operation with a 200% mortality risk. Lillehei had the strength of character to go ahead with 45 consecutive cases, correcting some of the most complicated congenital cardiac malformations. In 1955, after one of his presentations for correction of complicated tetralogy and pentology malformations,

Alfred Blalock said "I must say that I never thought I would see the day when this type of operative procedure could be performed. I want to commend Drs. Lillehei and Varco for their imagination, their courage and their industry". In closing the discussion Lillehei announced a bright future for the artificial oxygenator but not for the complex types that had been available to that time.

Just 16 days later on May 13 1955 Lillehei made his prediction come true by the first clinical use of the 'Lillehei-DeWall bubble oxygenator". Walt Lillehei felt that the complexity of the early heart-lung machine made the goal of safe bypass difficult. In 1955 Dr DeWall solved the problem of artificial bubble oxygenation utilizing 'Antifoam A and a helical reservoir. This achieved universal success and acceptance until the arrival of the disposable silastic membrane oxygenator years later. Many continued to use the screen method of the original gibbon design but it was more complicated. DeWall was a 27 year old General Practitioner turned researcher with the job of building a bubble oxygenator to be used instead of the cross-circulation donor. DeWall solved all the problems, the physiological ones such as large bubbles versus small ones as well as the practical ones. This turned out to be the prototype for the commercially produced disposable "Helix bubble oxygenator", enabling most of the early teams all over the world to finally embark on unhurried open-heart surgery. In 1954-1955 there were only two places, and two surgeons Lillehei and Kirklin performing open heart surgery since the cardio-pulmonary by-pass every thing became possible and spectacular accomplishments by new pioneers were still to come. First the heart valves by Hufnagel, Harken, Starr, and Lillehei himself, then the spectacular explosion of aorto-coronary bypass and finally transplantation by Barnard and Shumway – both trained by Walt Lillehei.

C. Walton Lillehei was able to tackle the problem before everybody else for two reasons. First the Wangensteen Clinic had a very strong laboratory and research base and having obtained a PhD, Lillehei was able to put together a very strong team for the open-heart surgery program. This team he was able to assemble played a crucial role in the ultimate success of the cross-circulation experiment and the first reliable bypass machine and the famous DeWall-Lillehi bubble oxygenator. Lillehei still worked in the laboratory when Morely Cohen, a young Canadian surgeon, joined him. Shortly there after they discovered the publication of Andreasen describing the low-flow 'azygos principle'. Morely Cohen with another student Herbert Warden performed all the experiments with the 'azygos principle' until he was ready to take the cross-circulation to the operating room. Richard DeWall only appeared for the bubble oxygenator which allowed the Lillehei team to progress from cross-circulation to the very first heart-lung machine functioning with DeWall at the machine in human case after human case.

Richard Varco was Lillehei's senior by 6 years and was one of Wagensteen's first residents. He was involved in every stage of early cardiovascular surgery in Minneapolis. Among the first surgeons to perform the Blalock operation outside of Johns Hopkins, he early on reported enviable results with the blue baby operation. He helped Clarence Dennis with his unfortunately unsuccessful operations using cardio-pulmonary bypass in 1951 and John Lewis with his first successful ASD closure under hypothermia and personally demonstrated the feasibility of operating for pulmonary stenosis under normothermic inflow occlusion. He encouraged Lillehei's work from the start and was his first assistant in all 45 cross-circulation cases. His moral support and help was an important factor in the ultimate acceptance of cross circulation.

SURGICAL PROCEDURES IN WHICH CARDIO-PULMONARY BYPASS IS USED

- Coronary bypass surgery
- Cardiac valve repair or replacement of any valve
- Repair of large septal defects
- Repair of / or palliation of congenital heart defects (tetrologyof Fallot, transposition of great vessels)
- Repair of some large aneurysms of the aorta
- Pulmonary thromboendarterectomy
- Pulmonary thrombectomy

History: Clarence Dennis led the team that conducted the first known operation involving open cardiotomy with temporary takeover of both heart and lungs functions on April 5, 1951 at the University of Minnesota Hospital, however the patient did not survive. In 1951 Dr. William T. Mustard cardiac surgeon at the hospital for Sick Children developed a heart-lung machine which permitted surgeons to open the hearts of living patients. But it was Gibbon who reported the first successful use of a heart-lung machine to repair a large atrial septal defect on May 6, 1953. Cardio-pulmonary bypass is designed so that it controls circulation and oxygenation on a temporary basis but it is also designed for inducing total body hypothermia so that circulation can be interrupted for a short period if needed. During open heart when there is no circulation to the heart myocardial hypothermia can be induced by bathing the heart in ice cold saline solution or by perfusing the coronary arteries with cold blood. Coronary artery perfusion is also a way to stop the heart by using a cold potassium solution. With resumption of coarse ventricular fibrillation and coronary perfusion at the completion of the intracardiac surgery the heart is easily restored to normal rythm by electrical defibrillation.

CHAPTER 5

Mininally Invasive Cardiac Surgery

MINIMALLY INVASIVE CARDIAC surgery (or robotics) has experienced a meteoric rise since its development in the 1990s. The first thoracic aortic stent graft was placed in July 1992, at Stanford University. Five years later, the Stanford group published their approach to mitral valve surgery through a right anterior thoracotomy, Alan Carpentier performed the first robotic assisted mitral valve operation. There has been an explosion of new techniques broadening the thoracic surgeon's armamentarium far beyond the typical median sternotomy and occasional left thoracotomy. While many of these techniques will become historical footnotes it is clear that minimally invasive cardiac surgery is here to stay, as 20% of mitral repairs are performed with some element of minimally invasive technique. Similarly thoracic endovascular aortic repair has become a well established treatment for aneurysmal disease and dissection of the thoracic aorta and is rapidly catching up with open repair as the treatment of choice.

Training has also changed. The last decade brought a surge of applications to traditional fellowship programs and the integrated thoracic surgery programs graduated their first trainees last year. With the variety of new operations and new techniques, novel training formats and professional goals for cardio-thoracic surgery trainees, how can we be sure that young cardiac surgeons are learning the skills they need to succeed in the coming decades. This includes open valve and coronary surgery on the heart side, while for thoracic surgery this includes traditional lung and esophageal resection, chest wall and pleural operations and importantly the widely practiced VATS lobectomy. The VATS lobectomy has been a recent but well received addition to the expected repertoire of graduates. The Board doesn't require mastery of any specific minimally invasive cardiac operation by the end of training but it does require that residents are exposed to a number of different endovascular and non-traditional approaches to coronary, valve and aortic surgery. The safety and efficacy of thoracic aortic stent grafting and minimally invasive mital surgery have already been proven to some degree. Teaching these new minimally invasive techniques is difficult because of lack of visualization for two people and controlling technical complications in a limited field. Because of the highly specialized nature of the operation, the relatively smaller patient base and the technical difficulty involved, it is often up to the highly motivated fellow or resident to gravitate to these repairs and seek out training on their own. Simulation training may be an important step to the goal of obtaining training in these advanced techniques and gathering experience functioning in the small space required of the operator. The resident will have to master the open operations and control of possible complications before accepting the responsibility that comes with robotics and working in tiny lonely spaces.

Types of valves

Valve replacement

PERSPECTIVES OF THORACIC SURGERY

The story of the replacement valves of the heart is long and complicated if done in its entirety and certainly is a tribute to the courage as well as the ingenuity of the men working in this field. There were deaths and complications as as might be expected in a group of patients with some very complicated lesions some close to death, some with associated lesions, some with multiple lesions requiring multiple valves and many with other types of disease affecting the heart such as coronary artery disease. The cloth-covered valve showed a markedly reduced incidence of thromboembolism even without anticoagulation. The incidence of thromboembolism without anticoagulation can be reduced to 1% with this design. This of course can be a great advantage to those who cannot tolerate any form of anticoagulation. Systolic gradients do vary with the the size of the valve which is dictated by orificial opening. The disc valve with cage has also received extensive trial on the premise that it produces more favorable hemodynamics with a larger frustrum area but this has not proven to be true. Valves with silastic or Teflon discs have shown a significant incidence of wear which restricts their use. The tilting disc valve originally introduced by Wada was subsequently redesigned by and imtroduced by Bjork in 1969. It has the advantage of a very low profile, a central flow concept, free floating lens without a cage and an extremely favorable ratio of inlet orifice and to mounting ring. As a result this valve has excellent hemodynamic function in smaller sizes. Peak systolic pressure and gradients across an aortic valve may vary depending on size and also on the location and design. It averaged 12.5 mm for the Bjork-Shiley, 17.5mm for the Starr Edwards and 27mm for the Kay-Shiley. Gradients become important for small aortic roots. The unstented homograft valves may present the best hemodynamics. Mortality rates are always significant information however there are so many variables in any one group that it is hard information to evaluate. Early mortality for the Starr-Edwards prosthesis for a variety of reports from the literature varied from 1.4to 10.8% and late mortality varied from 2.3 to 24 per cent. The greatest attrition happens during the first 12 to 18 months after operation. After that the course is more normal. In 1969 Bloodwell reported using a variety of caged ball valves in his long-term patients with a cumulative mortality of 26% after 7 years of followup. The problems that arose were myocardial failure, coronary insufficiency, arrhythmia, thromboembolism. Early and late deaths were usually the result of myocardial failure, coronary insufficiency, arrythmias, thrombo embolism, mechanical failure of the prosthesis, bacterial endocarditis, and cerebrovascular accidents.

Valve design

The designs were amazingly similar. They were ball valves with hollow metal balls in a metal usually cloth covered cage. There is a story for the cloth covering because it was soon noticed that though they functioned well and did the job they were prone to develop clot and produce a certain percentage of embolization and possible serious complications. The cloth covering the base and struts was used to develop a clot resisting surface that worked amazingly well.

TYPES OF HEART VALVES

There are two types of artificial heart valves, mechanical and tissue valves.

Tissue heart valves are usually made from animal tissue such as animal heart valves or animal pericardial tissue. The tissue is usually treated to prevent rejection and calcification. An alternative to animal tissue is a homograft valve usually a human aortic valve. The durability of a homograft valve is comparable to porcine or bovine tissue valves. Another method for procuring an aortic valve for replacement of a diseased aortic valve is the Ross procedure, which is to use the patient's own pulmonary valve to replace the aortic valve (an autograft valve) and then replace the pulmonary valve with a homograft valve (taken from another human at autopsy). This procedure was first used in 1967 and is primarily used in children. The advantages of this technique is that it eliminates rejection of the aortic valve because it is the patients own tissue and allows for growth in the child.

Mechanical valves are designed to outlast the patient. Although the mechanical valves (example is the ball valve for aortic stenosis or mitral insufficiency) are long lasting there is an increased risk of blood clots. As a result the recipient must take anticoagulants such as Warfarin for the rest of their lives. Tissue valves tend to wear out faster than mechanical valves particularly with increased flows as in a more active younger person. This means another operation for replacement of the worn out valve. For this reason mechanical valves are often recommended for the younger patient. Replacing the aortic valve usually requires a long incision over the middle of the sternum and the heart-lung machine to provide circulation and oxygenation while the surgeon works on the valve. Transesophageal echocardiogram (an ultrasound of the heart done through the esophagus) can be used to verify that the valve is functioning properly. Pacing wires are usually put in place so that the heart can be paced should rhythm problems or heart block occur. The risk of death is quoted at 1-3% but this depends on the condition of the patient prior to the operation. Robotic assisted techniques are now playing an increased role in performing operations on the aortic and mitral valves and we will discuss this next.

Treatment of Valvular Disease with artificial valves

Mitral valve regurgitation

Rheumatic Heart disease is the most common cause of mitral valve insufficiency. Competence of the mitral valve depends on an integrated function of the mitral annulus, the valve leaflets, the chordae tendineae, the papillary muscles and the ventricular wall. Incompetence can be caused by abnormalities of any of these structures. Involvement of the leaflets by the rheumatic process causes shortening, rigidity, and retraction of the cusps. The chordae tendineae also become fibrotic and fused and shortened. Commissural fusion also occurs so that the cusps are held open and secondary calcification of the leaflets is common. The most common disease of rheumatic heart disease is rheumatic mitral insufficiency. Varying degrees of stenosis may coexist with mitral insufficiency. Calcification of the mitral valve and annulus in the elderly can be an important cause of regurgitation and is often associated with hypertension, aortic stenosis, diabetes, and chronic renal failure. Calcification may involve the entire annulus and project into the adjacent myocardium. Calcium may prevent leaflet coaptation and it may even invade the conduction system. In extreme cases severe congestive heart failure and pulmonary edema may require emergency treatment. The variety of pathology with mitral insufficiency is immence. Because of the variety of pathologic changes in mitral insufficiency it did not lend itself to finger fracture like mitral stenosis though the pioneers of heart surgery tried all the blind techniques using finger fracture, through the atrial appendage knives via the apical route, and sharp instruments through both routes. Obviously after these blind techniques the insufficiency in some cases was not improved and might be worse. Mitral insufficiency may also be found in patients with hypertrophic obstructive cardiomyopathy due to an enlarged and displaced papillary muscle which pushes the anterior mitral leaflet into the outflow tract during systole. The final cause of mitral regurgitation is ischemic heart disease. Valve incompetence can be either primary as a result of muscle dysfunction or secondary to generalized ventricular and annular dilatation. A spectrum of severity of regurgitation exists. These range from patients with mild papillary muscle dysfunction to congestive heart failure and pulmonary edema. Moderate to severe regurgitation can be tolerated for many years. Atrial fibrillation is common. Systemic emboli can occur but not as common as in mitral stenosis. Bacterial endocarditis should be suspected with symptoms of malaise, fever and chills. The physical signs of congestive heart failure are similar to those found in mitral stenosis. The electrocardiogram may show ventricular hypertrophy. Biventricular and biatrial enlargement on x-ray can exhibit the greatest cardiomegaly of any valvular disease. Cardiac Catheterization reveals prominent left-atrial v- waves. With severe congestive failure left-ventricular end-diastolic pressure is elevated. Pulmonary hypertension has the same prognostic implications as in mitral stenosis. Patients with mild regurge may remain stable for years unless chordal rupture or infective endocarditis intervenes. After the appearance of heart failure the clinical status will deteriorate rapidly.

Surgical intervention is recommended for patients whose symptoms significantly limit life style or those in NYHA class III or IV congestive heart failure. The selection of operation procedure is where the difference from mitral stenosis comes in. Here-in comes the fine art of decision making. We have already indicated that the blind techniques through the apex of the right ventricle or the atrial appendage with the finger or instrument are not a satisfactory approach to the problem. We must now choose an open direct-vision approach with the options of attempting corrective surgery on the valve, on the fused chordae or even on distorted papillary muscles or annulus or should we excise the valve and replace it with a totally artificial valve, one of many that are now available. The selection of a valve for replacement will be influenced by the surgeons own preference and certainly by the results published by other surgeons. It is probable that longevity is improved after valve replacement though this opens up the list of possible valve complications such as embolization or the need for anticoagulation or for the low possibility of valve dysfunction. Operative mortality will vary according to associated medical disease, the NYHA class, coronary artery disease, and the status of left ventricular function. Mitral regurgitation seems to carry a poorer prognosis than mitral stenosis. Treatment as an emergency operation carries a higher mortality. The overall mortality for elective isolated mitral valve replacement is 2 to 5 per cent in most centers. But the technique-is still the surgeons choice. There is a group that favors a technique that favors what is called Minimally Invasive Mitral Valve Surgery which in general means a right thoracotomy with limited lower sternal division which may be less stressful for the patient with perhaps less recovery time.

We should also cover mitral valve repair without replacing the valve. Repair procedures include chordal and papillary muscle splitting, secondary chordal division, mitral ring annuloplasty, commissurotomy, chordal replacement, posterior leaflet extension, annular decalcification, and quadrangular resection. Secondary procedures include tricuspid ring annuloplasty, obliteration of left atrial appendage, left atrial ablation, left atrial reduction.

Tricuspid valve disease often is associated with mitral insufficiency. It usually presents as insufficiency and can be corrected by ring annuloplasty. Bakir et al repotrted their experience with mitral valve repair in 60 patients with an early mortality of 1.7%. Followup echocardiography revealed minimal or no mitral regurgitation in 35.5% and mild (1+) mitral regurge in 49%. Only 1 patient presented with severe mitral regurge post op. Left ventricular end diastolic diameter and left atrial diameter significantly decreased postop. Dr. Rakesh m. Suri from the Mayo Clinic reports that in patients with mitral valve regurgitation due to flail leaflets early surgery yields better survival, lower risk of heart failure and equivalent rates of atrial fibrillation. Over all long-term mortality is approximately 40% lower and heart failure risk approximately 60% lower for early surgery versus watchful waiting. The benefits persist up to 20 years and are seen across every subgroup of patients. These are the findings of a series of analyses of data from an international registry of consecutive patients diagnosed in routine clinical practice the largest study in the world of comparative effectiveness. Those who support watchful waiting feel that if the patient has not heart failure and has an ejection fraction 60% or more and a left ventricular endsystolic pressure of 40 mm or more consider the consequences of uncorrected mitral regurgitation to be benign. North American guidelines favor early surgery while European guidelines favor watchful waiting.

To end this discussion of mitral regurgitation we need to point out that children and infants also may suffer from mitral regurgitation and recently there is a report from Boston Children's Hospital describing a mitral replacement valve that may grow with the infant. There is the opportunity of sequential expansion as the child grows. It is called the Melody valve. Mechanical or prosthetic valves have a fixed size and must be replaced at the appropriate time. This new valve fills a gap in the availability of small valves and it is an externally stented bovine jugular vein graft that was designed for transcatheter pulmonary valve replacement. The valve in this study was inserted surgically. The valve maintains competence over a range of sizes up to 22 mm. The hope is that this valve can be enlarged in the catheterization laboratory as the child grows.

TAVR TRANSVENTRICULAR AORTIC VALVE REPLACEMENT

TAVR is a percutaneous approach to replacement of the aortic valve in elderly patients with severe symptomatic aortic stenosis ineligible for surgery because of high periperative risk. Usually this is a trans-femoral artery approach. Known as trans-catheter aortic valve implantation in a nonagenarian patient with severe symptomatic aortic stenosis. Open aortic valve surgery usually with replacement of the valve with a prosthesis has been described previously. There are a number of models to choose from depending on your experience and the experience of others. We now come to a class of patients that need a valve because they have symptomatic aortic stenosis but are not candidates for the open direct vision form of surgery usually because of age. The trans- catheter aortic valve implantation (TAVI) introduced by Cribier and colleagues in 2002, followed by a refinement of TAVI to a transfemoral approach by WEBB and co- workers in 2005 has challenged the idea that these high -risk patients are inoperable. The Sapiens trans - catheter valve has been designed to be introduced and placed in the aortic valve area using a trans femoral artery approach without the need for an incision in the chest that the standard aortic valve replacement would require. It is gaining in numbers of applications as experience is gained and designs change. This high risk stratum of patients now constitute about 10% of all patients needing an aortic valve. The Society of Thoracic Surgeon risk score is less than 4%. The Food and Drug administration has approved the Sapiens valve system. Patients given a choice favor the Sapien valve (TAVR) over the standard (SAVR) system because it is less invasive. The small number of high risk patients who go to open surgery tend to be men if their life expectancy is greater than 5-8 years or are patients with a high stroke risk (taken from a talk by Dr. Friedrich-Wilhelm Mohr). There is a transapical approach being tested but this has not been approved for general use. There is an increased risk for major vascular complications and for stroke during the the first month post implant. We should note that there is a trans catheter mitral valve repair study in progress but it is too early for comments or predictions.

    In 2013 a report after I year of the over all survival with the transcatheter aortic Core valve in the post market ADVANCE study was 82.1% and cardiovascular survival was 88.2%. This compares with survival rates of 87.4% at 6months and 95.5% at 30 days. If we look at the PARTNER A and B cohorts in the pivotal trial in the SAPIEN transcatheter valve system the mortality rate was 8 to 13% lower. One explanation is that the 1,015 patient study sought out centers experienced with transcatheter aortic valve implantation (TAVI). The 44 centers in Western Europe, Asia, and South America had to have performed at least 40 TAVI procedures, with some German centers having done at least 500, to be certified by a TAVI proctor and to have a heart team in place. In comparison some centers in the PARTNER trial of the Edwards Lifesciences Sapien study contributed just six or seven patients and were selected based on their experience with general cardiologic intervention.

The 1 year survival rates in ADVANCE also surpass those of early registries., notably the French Aortic National Core Valve and Edwards registry where the initial experience with TAVI was associated with interventional mistakes which were linked to early mortality. The Core Valve System has been implanted in more than 30,000 patients since approval in the European Union in 2007, but is limited to investigational use in the United States.

There are no details about mortality in various subgroups or complications such as stroke, paravalvular leaks, or left bundle branch block (LBBB) after TAVI with a balloon expandable valve. A recent analysis raised concerns about LBBB showing that 1/3 of 202 consecutive patients with no prior conduction problems developed new onset LBBB after TAVI with a balloon expandible valve such as SAPIEN or SAPIEN XT. Although it resolved in 37% by hospital discharge and 57% by 6 to 12 months, this group had a significantly higher incidence of syncope, and complete atrioventricular block requiring a permanent pacemaker. There has been no evidence of a problem with LBBB in an early followup in ADVANCE. Quality of life data from Advance showed significant benefits with COREVALVE even in higher risk patients. The Food and Drug Administration has expanded Approval for the SAPIEN transcatheter heart valve for patients with aortic stenosis who are at high risk for serious surgical complications or death. The transapical approach was not approved outside of clinical trials. It requires insertion through the ribs and the through the apical myocardium. STS has launched an investigational study with the American College of Cardiology that may allow more patients to benefit from transcatheter aortic valve. TAVR using the EDWARDS SAPIEN valve was recently approved in the United States for inoperable or high risk patients with aortic stenosis. Some patients have too much disease in the femoral artery to permit the current approach. The new study will evaluate the safety and efficacy of alternative access routes for TAVR, including transapical, transaortic, transsubclavian, transaxillary, and transiliac. An estimated 1 in4 patients have been ineligible for TAVR because advanced disease precludes use of the FDA approved access site.

The CORE VALVE for transcatheter aortic valve replacement in patients with severe aortic stenosis at increased surgical risk was found superior to surgical valve replacement showing a significantly lower risk of mortality 1 year later. In the U.S. CORE VALVE High Risk study, a prospective randomized controlled study of almost 800 patients, the rate of all-cause mortality at one year was 14.2% among those in the transcatheter aortic valve replacement group (TAVR) compared with 19.1% among those in the surgery group, a significant difference. This is the first prospective randomized study to show superiority for the transcatheter valve therapy over surgery. Based on these studies TAVR may become the alternative of choice for patients at this level of risk. The CORE VALVE self-expanding prosthesis was approved in January 2014 by the Food and Drug Administration for use in extreme risk patients. The effect of TAVR using the CORE VALVE device was compared to 795 patients at 45 U.S. centers. The patients had severe aortic stenosis, Class II heart failure or higher and were judged to have at least a risk of 15% risk of death within 30 days after surgery. Mean age was 83. And almost half were female. Other risk factors included coronary artery disease (in about 2/3), previous coronary bypass surgery (about 30%), a previous myocardial infaction(about 25%) and almost all had heart failure. Permanent Pacemaker implantations were significantly higher in the TAVR group (22.3% at 1 year vs 11.3% in the surgical group). In the TAVR group there were 5 cases of perforations whereas there were no cases of perforation in the surgical group. In the SAPIEN AORTIC TRANSCATHETER group in high risk patients with severe aortic stenosis there was no difference in mortality between the two and an increase in cerebrovascular events in the TAVR arm.

There is a study for transcatheter mitral valve repair for mitral regurgitation. Two devices show promise though it is believed to be primarily a surgical problem. Two devices are relevant to these indications though neither is yet approved by the Food and Drug Administration. These are Cardiac Dimensions CARILLON for annular dilatation and Abbott Vascular's MITRACLIP for leaflet repair. In the European TITAN clinical trial, 36 of 53 patients (68%) demonstrated were implanted with the CARILLON Mitral Contour System. The average baseline ejection fraction of all 53 patients was 28% characterized as true mitral regurgitation. The non-randomized double- arm study compared results from the implanted group to results from a group without implants. The implanted patients demonstrated significant reductions in mitral regurgitation. These and other measures correlated with symptomatic improvement. The other device, the MitraClip was evaluated in the EVEREST II trial for safety and efficacy in the treatment of mitral valve regurgitation. The primary effectiveness defined by the trial showed surgery as more effective. MitraClip is not being used for low-risk patients amenable to surgical repair. However those patients who did have a good result with MITRCLIP, the results seem to be durable. There is a new trial underway called the COAPT trial which has been approved by the FDA. This is truly a trial looking at palliative benefit not mortality.

There is a new smaller version of the SAPIEN valve the only transcatheter aortic valve available for the U.S. use. This showed non-inferior results, and clinical outcomes and safer procedural results in a U.S. comparison of the new and existing devices raising expectations that the new valve system, the SAPIEN XT, will soon be on the market. Although the new SAPIEN valve matches the former model in the incidence of important adverse effects of residual or moderate or even severe parabasilar leaks, several U.S operators who perform transcatheter aortic valve repair (TAVR) stress that the leak problem has begun to resolve recently as surgeons have found ways to minimize the issue. Patients treated with the new XT version of the SAPIEN VALVE had significantly fewer procedural complications, fewer major vascular events, (10% with the XT device, compared with 16% with the approved valve) and significantly fewer disabling bleeding events (8% with the XT device, compared with 13% with the first generation system). Patients treated with the XT device also required significantly fewer episodes when initially placed valve had to be replaced and fewer aborted procedures (two compared with eight using the approved valve). The new valve required an average of 14 minutes less anesthesia time, a significant difference. The big concerns from the first PARTNER trial were vascular complications, strokes, and paravascular leaks. The vascular complications were reduced and the stroke rate went down.

But there is even more. Though the valves could now be placed with all its complicated aspects many patients were not eligible because of other problems such as intolerance of drugs, previous surgery etc. A new technique is finding its way into the lexicon and the dictionary of new procedures called transcatheter aortic valve replacement. Aortic valve disease is commonly treated by now by aortic valve replacement but the open procedure is considererd dangerous for high risk patients with multiple organ dysfunction. Approximately 30% to 40% of elderly patients with severe, symptomatic aortic valve stenosis are deemed ineligible because of high perioperative risk. Transcatheter aortic valve replacement has been developed as an alternative technique for just such a group. The convential surgery is not an option for patients of advanced age. If left untreated aortic stenosis is a rapidly progressive disease with a mortality of approximately of 50% in the first 2 years. Approximately 30-40% of elderly patients with severe symptomatic valve stenosis are deemed ineligible for surgery because of high perioperative risk. However the intrduction of a percutaneous approach by Cribier in 2002 followed by a refinement to a transfemoral approach by Webb and and associates in 2005, has challenged the idea that these high risk patients are inoperable. Trans femoral [TAVI] is the only therapy that has been associated in a randomized trial with survival rates equivalent or superior to those of surgical experience in europe. In elderly patients the aortic valve as well as the aorta is often heavily calcified and brittle which poses a risk because manipulation often dislodges calcium and may cause a stroke. TAVI is less invasive and offers a lower mortality risk. The true stroke risk is still being evaluated. Kneitz etal report a case of a 90 year woman diagnosed with severe aortic stenosis aggravated by physical activity she had a history of hypertension chronic obstructive disease hypothyroidism, congestive heart failure, atrial fibrillation and renal insufficiency. She had undergone pacemaker implantation for sinoatrial ablation. At age 95 she had dyspnea with minmal exertion. She could no longer walk. An open procedure was too risky She developed shortness of breath aggravated by physical activity and could only walk 20 feet. She gave consent to having TAVI and three weeks later had only mild shortness of breath on exertion and could walk 10 to 15 feet at at a time and walk to a cafeteria. This did not alter the course of the aortic stenosis. Thus here is a procedure that while it does not add years to your life if candidates are carefully selected it can dramatically improve the patients life. The alternative access to using the femoral access that has been described still remains to be proven and accepted. Some patients have too much disease in the femoral artery to permit the femoral approach. A new study will test an alternative approach for TAVR includimg the apex of the heart, the aorta and the transaxillary and trans subclavian arteries. An estimated 1 in 4 patients are ineligible because of advanced disease at the approved access site and Fred Edwards MD will determine whether alternative access procedures will work. New clinical guidelines will be developed to make recommendations in 26 areas including mechanical valves and biological valves.

CARPENTIER MITRAL VALVE

After following more than 400 patients who underwent mitral valve replacement for almost 25 years, French investigators have found that the Carpentier- Edwards Perimount Pericardial prosthetic has an expected durability of more than 16 years with a low incidence of valve-related complications. In this prospective study investigators found 404 patients who underwent mitral valve replacement between August 1984 to March 2011; 46 of these patients eventually needed a second bioprosthesis. Patients were asked to complete yearly clinical questionaires and undergo an echocardiographic study. Their mean age was 68 years, but the range was 22-89 years. Amost one fourth of the group was age 60 or younger. The mean followup time was 7.2 years though it ranged from 0 to 24years. Ten patients were lost to followup yielding a 98% completion rate. Fifty–seven per cent were New York Heart Association class III or IV. The operative mortality was 3.3%. A total of 188 patients had late death. Forty of the deaths were valve related including 5 due to thromboembolism, 4 due to endocarditis, 4 due to structural valve dysfunction and 23 to sudden death. Valve related survival was more than 60% at 20 years post surgery. Valve related events were rare including endocarditis, thromboembolism and bleeding. There were no cases of valve thrombosis. Seventy-six patients had severe mitral regurgitation even if patients were asymptomatic. Of these 63 were reoperated and 13 died before reoperation. Three quarters of the valves failed due to calcification while 20% had late leaflet tears and 4% had mixed problems. For the entire group it took an average of 16.6 years before a severe valvular defect occurred although freedom from SVD (structural valve dysfunction) differed according to age at surgery. Older patients fared better. After 16.6 years, 75% of those over 70 were expected to be free from SVD while the rates were lower for those between 60 and 70 years (52%) and those under age 60 (40%). The author's report felt that the Carpentier-Edwards valve was a reliable choice for patients older than 60. Patients under age 60 still receive mechanical valves of which Starr-Edwards valve is an example.

Adendum to section on surgical treatment of dangerous and/or uncontrollable rythm disturbances that do not respond to medical therapy.

THIS IS ADDED AS AN ADDENDUM NOT SO MUCH TO TEACH CARDIOLOGY BUT TO ILLUSTRATE CHANGES AND ADDITIONS TO OUR KNOWLEDGE NOT ONLY OF CARDIOLOGY BUT ALSO THE INCREASING ROLE THAT SURGERY NOW PLAYS IN THE TREATMENT WHAT USED TO BE ONLY A CARDIOLOGY PROBLEM. THE ARRYTHMIAS USED TO BE TREATED WITH MEDICATIONS AND SYNCHRONIZED ELECTRIC SHOCKS. SOME WITH SUCCESS BUT NOT ALWAYS. NOW THERE IS A WHOLE BODY OF SURGICAL PROCEDURES THAT CAN BE RESORTED TO WHEN MEDICATION AND ELECTRICAL TOOLS DON'T WORK. THE ANATOMY AND THE INSTRMENTATION HAVE CHANGED AND BECOME MORE SOPHISTICATED BUT OUR KNOWLEDGE OF THE ANATOMY AND FUNCTION OF THE CONDUCTION SYSTEM AS WELL AS THE ABNORMALITIES OF THE CONDUCTION SYSTEM HAVE IMPROVED REMARKABLY TO THE POINT THAT SOME CAN NOW BE TREATED SURGICALLY. THE DISCUSSION OF ABNORMAL AND DANGEROUS RYTHMS IS NOT INTENDED TO MAKE ANYONE AN EXPERT BUT ONLY TO INFORM YOU OF THE EXISTENCE OF CERTAIN SURGICAL TREATMENT OPTIONS FOR WHAT HAS ALWAYS BEEN A PROBLEM FOR CARDIOLOGISTS AND OFTEN MEDICALLY INSOLUBLE. IT IS A COMPLICATED SUBJECT EVEN FOR MOST THORACIC AND CARDIAC SURGEONS.

CHAPTER 6

Cardiac Arrhythmias, Surgical Treatment

SURGERY HAS BECOME an acceptable treatment for some cardiac intractable arrhythmias. Several innovative surgical techniques have been introduced for the treatment of supraventricular tachycardia due to Wolff- Parkinson-White (WPW) Syndrome, concealed accessory atrio-ventricular connections, A-V node reentry tachycardia, ectopic (automatic) atrial tachycardia, atrial flutter fibrillation, and both ischemic and non-ischemic ventricular tachyarrythmias.

The sinoatrial node is a small subepicardial group of highly specialized cells located in the sulcus terminalis just lateral to the junction of the superior vena cava and the right atrium. The cells are arranged around a central SA node artery that may arise from either the right or left coronary system and may pass either anterior or posterior to the superior vena cava. Studies suggest that the SA node consists of three distinct regions each responsive to a separate group of neural and circulatory stimuli. The interrelationship of these regions determines the ultimate output of the SA node. Under normal conditions, these cells are the only ones in the heart that are capable of spontaneous Phase 4 depolarization thus establishing the SA node as the site of origin of the normal cardiac impulse. The existence of specialized conduction pathways between the SA node and the atrioventricular node (AV) has been the subject of controversy. Most authorities now agree that while an electrical impulse emanating from the SA node travels to the AV node preferentially via the crista terminalis and the limbus of the fossa ovalis these muscle bundles do not represent specialized insulated conduction tracts comparable to the ventricular bundle branches. Although electrical impulses travel more rapidly through these thick atrial muscle bundles surgical transection will not block internodal conduction. The atrioventricular junctional area is the most complex anatomic portion of the cardiac conduction system. From a functional standpoint, the A-V node should be considered as the area in which a normal delay in atrioventricular conduction occurs. This area corresponds anatomically to a group of atrioventricular junctional cells that are histologically distinct from working myocardium. As an atrial impulse approaches the AV node area, it traverses a transition zone of specialized cells located anteriorly in the base of the atrial septum slightly to the right of and cephalad to the central fibrous body. This transition zone surrounds the atrial aspect of the compact atrial node where the major conduction delay occurs. The lower longitudinal portion of the compact AV node penetrates the central fibrous body immediately posterior to the membranous portion of the interatrial septum to become the bundle of His. The AV node, its transitional zone, and its penetrating bundle within the triangle of Koch, an anatomically discreet region is bounded by the tendon of Todaro, the tricuspid valve annulus and the thebesian valve of the coronary sinus. There is little danger of surgical damage to the AV conduction if all procedures avoid this triangle. Once the penetrating portion of the AV node traverses the central fibrous body it becomes the bundle of His. The annulus of the tricuspid valve is situated more toward the ventricular apex than is that of the mitral valve. The bundle of His courses along the posterior inferior rim of the membranous portion of the interventricular septum. The right bundle branch proceeds subendocardially towards the ventricular apex in the intra-myocardial substance of the trabeculae of the septomarginalis and ramifies at the apex, partly crossing the cavity of the ventricle in the moderator band. At the lower level of the membranous interventricular septum the His bundle gives off a broad band of fasciculi forming the left bundle branch that extends down the left side of the septum for a distance of one to two cm. where it divides into a smaller anterior and a larger posterior radiation. The medial aspect of each of these radiations usually become intermeshed distally to form three anastomosing nets of fibers: anterior, middle and posterior.

The danger area from the standpoint of of the conduction tissue is immediately subjacent to the right coronary-noncoronary commissure.

The distal branches of the conduction system terminate in an intermediate zone between the Purkinj cells and the myocardium, where the cells gradually lose their Purkinje characteristics and take on the characteristics of of working ventricular myocardium. Of particular importance to the cardiac surgeon dealing with conduction abnormalities are the relationships of the various structures and potential spaces comprising the junction of the atrial septum, the ventricular septum atrio-ventricular grooves and the fibrous skeleton of the heart. The cardiac skeleton of the heart is strongest at the central fibrous body where the annuli of the mitral, aortic and tricuspid valves meet. Since the tricuspid annulus is more apical in position than the mitral annulus, the anterior part of the central fibrous body extends into the ventricles beneath the attachment of the tricuspid valve and forms the interventricular component of the membranous septum between the aortic outflow tract and the right atrium. Likewise Immediately posterior to the membranous septum the right atrial wall is in potential communication with the inlet portion of the left ventricle. The mitral and aortic valve annuli contribute significantly to the structural integrity of the fibrous skeleton and are further strengthened to form the left fibrous trigone. The left anterior portion of the central fibrous body is designated as the right fibrous trigone. The AV groove between these two trigones represents the site of continuity between the anterior leaflet of the mitral valve and the aortic valve annulus and is the only area in the AV groove where atrial muscle is not in juxtaposition to ventricular muscle For this reason accessory atrioventricular pathways are not found between the left and right fibrous trigones. The potential space overlying the inlet septum has been demonstrated to harbor all posterior septal accessory pathways in the WPW syndrome. The floor of this pyramidal space is formed by the upper posterior interventricular septum. The space contains the terminal portion of the coronary sinus, the AV node artery and the fat pad. This complex anatomy is a challenge for any surgeon attempting to ablate an accessory AV connection passing through this space.

- The proper selection of patients for the surgical treatment of cardiac arrhythmias is based on a number of variables including

age, general condition, nature of presenting arrhythmia, its response to medical treatment and the presence of associated anomalies that may require surgical correction.
- Supraventricular Tachyarrhymias: preoperative electrophysiologic evaluation

  ➢ Atrial flutter
  ➢ Atrial fibrillation
  ➢ Junctional tachycardia
  ➢ Chaotic atrial tachycardia
  ➢ Sick sinus syndrome

These can be diagnosed by routine non-invasive electrocardiography However refractory supraventricular due to an accessory atrioventricular connection (WPW syndrome), enhanced AV node connection, AV node reentry, Mahaim fibers, or concealed accessory connections that conduct only retrograde require more sophisticated electrophysiologic evaluation. This requires catheters placed in the high right atrium, low right atrium, coronary sinus, (quadripolar catheter) right ventricular apex, and along the bundle of His. The initial His bundle recordings are helpful in determining whether or not an accessory pathway is present. Normally the His bundle recordings reveal atrial activity at the onset of the P wave and ventricular activity at the onset of the QRS complex of the standard electrocardiogram. If an accessory connection is present that bypasses the AV node, the A-H and the A-V intervals are shortened but the H-V interval is normal. This anomaly is classified clinically as the "enhanced AV node conduction" and if refactory to medical therapy it requires either endocardial catheter ablation or surgical cryoablation of both the accessory pathway and the His bundle since they usually cannot be separated anatomically at the time of surgery. In the presence of a Mahaim fiber connecting the His bundle to the septal myocardium, the A-H interval is normal because the electrical impulse is unaffected until after it exits the AV node. However the H-V interval is shortened because the impulse can travel via the Mahaim fiber to the myocardium resulting in pre-excitation and a delta wave. When a complete atrioventricular bypass tract exists (Kent bundle in the WPW syndrome) the electrical impulse travels both antegrade down the normal conduction system (normal A-H interval) and antegrade down the Kent bundle (markedly shortened A-V interval) This results in pre-excitation of the ventricular myocardium at the site of insertion of the Kent bundle, producing the short PR interval, delta wave, and wide QRS complex characteristic of the WPW syndrome. It may be difficult to differentiate between AV node re-entry and the WPW syndrome if stable ante-grade pre-excitation does not exist. In these cases, the patient undergoes programmed electrical stimulation of the atrium in an effort to induce reciprocating tachycardia. Once stable tachycardia is induced a premature ventricular stimulus is delivered immediately after activation of the His bundle. If the atrium is pre-excited by the premature ventricular stimulus, an accessory pathway capable of retrograde conduction must be present, because retrograde conduction up the His bundle would be impossible because of its state of refractoriness. Inability to pre-excite the atrium by introducing a premature ventricular stimulus during induced supraventricular tachycardia is strong evidence for the presence of AV node re-entry. If the patient has refractory supraventricular tachy cardia due to AV node reentry, several surgical approaches may be possible, including endocardial catheter ablation of the His bundle, surgical cryoablation of the bundle of His, and discrete cryosurgery of the AV node.

If an accessory AV connection is documented by the above techniques an effort is made to determine the location because the surgical approach to left free-wall and right free-wall and septal pathways is different. In addition accessory AV connections occasionally become non-functional at the time of surgery due to trauma or anesthesia, precluding intraperative localization of the site of the accessory pathway. Free-wall left-sided pathways are identified primarily by two means (1) during induced reciprocating tachycardia or ventricular pacing, the quadripolar coronary sinus catheter (which is in contact with the posterior left atrial wall) records atrial activity travelling retrograde across the accessory pathway earlier than do the right atrial catheters and (2) by inducing left bundle branch block (LBBB) during reciprocating tachycardia, the V-A interval is prolonged 35 msec or more in the presence of a free-wall pathway. This prolongation of the V-A interval with LBBB occurs because normally during reciprocating tachycardia the impulse travels down the His bundle branch and left ventricular myocardium and retrograde up the left-sided accessory pathway to reach the atrium. However with LBBB the impulse must travel down the right bundle branch across the septum to the left ventricular myocardium and then up the accessory pathway to the atrium. The longer route results in significant prolongation of the V-A interval. The opposite electrophysiological findings occur in the presence of a right free-wall accessory pathway. Induced right bundle branch block (RBBB) during reciprocating tachycardia results in a prolongation of the V-A interval of 35 msec or more. Septal pathways are suspected if the V-A interval is not prolonged – i.e. prolonged less than 35 msec. with either RBBB or LBBB. In addition the proximal electrode on the quadripolar cononary sinus catheter is normally positioned at the coronary sinus orifice, and in the presence of a septal pathway it records the earliest atrial impulse during reciprocating tachycardia. Also a study of the functional properties of the accessory pathway and associated arrhythmias is accomplished by performing straight pacing as well as refractory period determinations from the right atrium, the left atrium (ie the coronary sinus), the right ventricle and rarely the left ventricle This allows assessment of the conduction and refractoriness of the normal conduction system and the accessory pathway in both antegrade and retrograde directions.

Wolff Parkinson White Syndrome

The description of the WPW syndrome as a distinct entity in 1930 prompted considerable controversy regarding the cause of the observed electrcardiographic abnormalities. The combination of a short P-R interval, delta wave and widened QRS complex was attributed to fusion beats, hyperexcitable myocardium in the upper ventricular septum, accelerated A-V node conduction, longitudinal dissociation in the His bundle, and accessory AV connections in or around the AV node but within the septum. Thus, direct surgical treatment of the WPW syndrome became feasible only after a conclusive demonstration that an abnormal anatomic connection existed between the atrium and ventricle and that this connection was capable of conducting electrical impulses. Holtzmann first suggested that the short PR interval and delta wave might result from early excitation of the ventricle by an impulse that passed via an accessory AV pathway. His theory was supported anatomically by the earlier studies of Kent who described muscular bridges connecting the right atrium and the right ventricle in a variety of mammalian species. In 1958 Truex demonstrated similar muscular bridges between the atrium and ventricle in human hearts up to the age of 6 months. In 1967 Durrer employed intraoperative epicardial mapping techniques to provide the first direct electrophysiologic evidence of ventricular pre-excitation occurring via an accessory AV connection in a patient with WPW syndrome. Also in 1967 Burchel confirmed Durrer's findings and was able to abolish ventricular pre-excitation temporarily by injecting procaine into the AV groove at the site of the earliest ventricular excitation. Final demonstration of the presence of functional accessory AV connections and their importance in the genesis of the WPW syndrome occurred in 1968 when Sealy surgically divided the accessory AV pathway in a patient with type B WPW syndrome. The procedure resulted in a normal P-R interval and QRS complex with disappearance of the delta wave and permanently abolished the ventricular pre-excitation and recurrent supraventricular tachyarrythmia. The surgical procedure for interruption of an accessory AV connection in the WPW syndrome consists of two steps (1) localization of the accessory pathway by intraoperative electrical mapping techniques and (2) division of the accessory pathway. After performing a median sternotomy fixed epicardial electrodes are sutured to both atrium and ventrical for purposes of pacing and recording. Generally the electrodes are positioned as close as possible to the suspected site of the accessory pathway. Epicardial unipolar electrograms recorded from normal human myocardium vary in amplitude from 20 to 60 mV on the ventricle and 2 to 10 mV on the atrium. Bipolar derivatives of closely spaced unipolar electrodes record amplitudes one half this value. Epicardial unipolar recordings are generally recorded at frequency settings of 0.1 to 1200 Hz. The low frequency response tends to make the the unipolar electrogram unstable but the bipolar derivative of two adjacent electrodes recorded at filter frequencies of 5.0 to 1200 Hz provides a sharp deflection ideally suited to trigger a digital timer.

In patients with the WPW syndrome the intraoperative mapping technique is performed as follows. If the patient is in normal sinus rhythm with stable antegrade pre-excitation, the initial electrophysiologic map is performed using a ventricular reference. This map localizes the site(s) of earliest ventricular activation, thereby establishing the location of the ventricular insertion of the accessory pathway. In patients in whom stable antegrade pre-excitation is not present at the beginning of the mapping study, the atrium is paced in a region near the suspected site of the accessory pathway to elicit ventricular pre-excitation. However, atrial pacing under these circumstances may obscure the possible detection of other accessory pathways by promoting preferential conduction across the nearest accessory AV connection. If stable antegrade pre-excitation cannot be elicited the accessory pathway can be localized by retrograde (atrial) mapping during reciprocating tachycardia or ventricular pacing. Many patients do not exibit stable reciprocating tachycardia during surgery whereas others may not tolerate the hemodynamic consequences associated with this arrhythmia. In this situation a retrograde (atrial) map during ventricular pacing near the suspected site of the accessary pathway will localize the accessory tract. This technique, however, may also obscure more remote accessoryAV connections. It is usually necessary to institute cardiopulmonary bypass in these patients to provide hemodynamic stability while performing retrograde mapping. Although the above steps are capable of localizing the accessory pathway in the majority of patients special problems may be encountered occasionally. In the presence of a septal accessory pathway the point of earliest epicardial excitation occurs at a site remote from the actual location of the accessory AV pathway. Therefore a surgical incision at the site of earliest epicardial ventricular activation will not modify the pre excitation. Fortunately certain features of the epicardial map may suggest the presence of a septal pathway. By recording unipolar epicardial data near the site of earliest excitation with free-wall AV connections, the earliest ventricular activation occurs before or simultaneously with the onset of the delta wave. In patients with septal pathways the earliest epicardial activation occurs after the onset of the surface delta wave. In most patients with either anterior or posterior septal pathways total cardiopulmonary bypass is instituted. Endocardial retrograde atrial mapping is performed following a right atriotomy to confirm the location of the septal pathway

Atrial fibrillation also constitutes a special problem because no stable antegrade pre-excitation can be established, and retrograde (atrial) mapping is impossible. This problem is circumvented by recording variable activation times between the ventricular reference electrode and any given ventricular site. By noting only those beats with early activation times and manifest pre-excitation, the site of ventricular insertion of the accessory atrioventricular connection can usually be identified.

Surgical Technique

Accessory AV connections may occur at any point around the annulus fibrosus on either side of the heart except that portion of the mitral valve annulus between the right and left fibrous trigones. However from a surgical standpoint, their locations are classified as right free-wall, left free-wall, anterior septal, or posterior septal. A median sternotomy is performed regardless of the suspected position of the accessory AV pathway prior to surgery. Once the atrial and ventricular insertions of the accessory pathway have been identified cardiopulmonary bypass is begun. If the pathway is located on the right side, the superior vena cava is cannulated via the deep femoral vein to allow better visualization of the right annulus fibrosus. The heart is arrested with cold potassium cardioplegic solution for the dissection of all accessory atrioventricular connections, and 2.5 optical magnification is used for all operative procedures. Accessory pathways on the right free-wall are approached initially by performing right atriotomy. The area of the annulus fibrosus corresponding to the site of the accessory AV connection is identified, and a supra-annular incision is placed approximately 2 mm above the annulus of the tricuspid valve exposing the AV groove fat pad encompassing the right coronary artery and vein. Generally, the incision is extended 2 cm on each side of the previously determined location of the accessory pathway. The AV groove fat pad containing the coronary vessels is separated from the top of the external wall of the ventricle all the way to the ventricular epicardial reflexion throughout the length of the supra—annular incision. All fibrous bands and small vessels are divided if they enter the ventricle. The extension of this incision anteromedially to the anterior aspect of the membranous septum is occasionally necessary in order to divide anterior septal pathways passing through the fat pad between the right fibrous trigone and the site of insertion of the right coronary into the AV groove. This fat pad lies just anterior to the membranous portion of the interatrial septum between the ascending aorta and the medial wall of the right atrium. After completion of the AV groove dissection a sharp nerve hook or knife divides any remaining fibers between the atrium and ventricle of the tricuspid valve annulus. This last maneuver allows visualization of the tricuspid valve annulus throughout the length of the supra-annular incision which is then closed with continuous non absorbable suture.

Exposure of left freewall pathways is accomplished via a left atiotomy in the manner used routinely to expose the mitral valve. All patients with left freewall pathways undergo the same surgical dissection regardless of the precise location of the pathway. A supra-annular incision is placed 2 mm above the posterior mitral valve annulus from the left fibrous trigone to the posterior interventricular septum. A plane of dissection is established between the underlying AV groove fat pad and the top of the posterior left ventricle throughout the length of the supra-annular incision. The plane of dissection is carried to the epicardium as it reflects off the posterior left ventricle onto the AV groove fat pad throughout the length of the supra-annular incision. A sharp nerve hook or knife divides any remaining fibers connecting the atrium to the ventricle at the level of the posterior mitral valve annulus, and the supra-annular incision is closed with a 4-0 non-absorbable suture. The most difficult accessory AV connections to interrupt surgically are located posteriorly in the region of the crux (posterior septal) pathways. A right atriotomy is performed in these patients prior to arresting the heart with cold potassium cardioplegia. The His bundle is identified with a hand held probe used to map the lower right interatrial septum. Once the His bundle is identified, a supra-annular incision just posterior to the site of the His bundle and extended in a counterclockwise direction onto the posterior right atrial free-wall. A plane of dissection is established between the fat pad and the top of the posterior interventricular septum. Dissection in the region of the His bundle is performed during either atrial pacing or reciprocating tachycardia to avoid injury to the AV node-His bundle complex. Once dissection has been completed the heart is arrested with cold potassium cardioplegic solution and the remainder of the posterior pyramidal space overlying the posterior interventricular septum is dissected. This dissection is carried medially to the level of the mitral valve annulus and posteriorly to the epicardial reflexion off the the posterior ventricular surface. Particular attention is paid to dissection of the left corner of the pyramidal space overlying the posterior superior process of the left ventricle at the site where the posterior interventricular septum is juxtaposed to the posterior free-wall of the left ventricle. After dissection the supra-annular incision is closed with a continuous 4-0 nonabsorbable suture.

Surgical Results

Between 1968 and May 20 1984 300 patients underwent elective surgical treatment for WPW syndrome at Duke University or at Barnes Hospital in St Louis. In the first 200 patients surgical division of the accessory atrioventricular pathway was successful in 98% of right free-wall pathways, 92% of left free-wall pathways and 77% of posterior septal pathways. A large percentage of these patients required two or more operations before the accessory pathway was divided successfully. In the last 100 patients, 131 of 132 (99.2%) accessory atrioventricular connections were divided successfully at the time of the first operation except in one patient with a right anterior free-wall pathway that was initially dissected from outside the heart without instituting cardiopulmonary bypass because of depressed function. Ventricular pre-excitation occurred immediately after surgery. The patient was returned to the operating room where a standard dissection was performed from the endocardium with successful division of the accesary connection. There have been no return of ventricular pre-excitation or of reciprocating tachycardia, and none of the patients have been treated with antiarryythmic medications for the WPW syndrome postoperatively. Thirty- nine posterior septal pathways encountered in the last 100 patients and all 39 were successfully divided surgically.

Paroxysmal Supraventricular Tachycardia Due to Concealed Accessory Atrioventricular Connections

Patients who have paroxysmal supraventricular tachycardia (PSVT) due to a concealed accessory atrioventricular connection that conducts in the retrograde (ventricular-atrial) direction only are approached surgically in the same manner that one approaches a patient with the standard WPW syndrome. Since the accessory atrioventricular connection in these patients is incapable of conducting in the antegrade (atrial–ventricular) direction no delta wave is present on the ECG during normal sinus rhythm and thus at the time of surgery, ventricular epicardial mapping is of no value. Retrograde atrial mapping is performed during induced reciprocating tachycardia or during ventricular pacing accessory to identify the site of atrial insertion of the accessory pathway, which is then divided surgically according to the methods described above.

Paroxysmal Supraventricular Tachycardia Due to AV Node Reentry

Prior to 1981, the only surgical therapy available for patients with medical refractory AV node re-entry tachycardia was elective cryoablation of the bundle of His. In this procedure an epicardial pacing electrode is sutured on the right atrium, and normothermic cardiopulmonary bypass is instituted. A right atriotomy is performed and a hand-held exploring electrode is positioned over the suspected site of the His bundle posteriorly to the membranous portion of the interatrial septum during atrial pacing. Once a definite His/complex is recorded by the handheld electrode the electrode is replaced wth a cryoprobe the tip of which can be cooled with internally expanding nitrous oxide. The cryoprobe temperature is decreased to 0 degrees C, at which time atrioventricular conduction should cease. The tissue is then allowed to rewarm to normothermia, at which time AV conduction returns. This temporary cooling and rewarming confirms that the tip of the cryoprobe is in the appropriate position overlying the His bundle. The temperature of the probe is then deceased to -60 degrees C for two minutes resulting in cryoablation of the His bundle and permanent atrio-ventricular conduction block. Thirty- one patients have undergone elective cryoablation of the bundle of His at Duke University for a variety of refractory supraventricular tachyarrhythmias with a success rate of 89%.

In 1981, a closed- chest technique was described for permanent His bundle ablation in which 200 to 500 joules are delivered through a His bundle catheter. This procedure has effectively replaced cryoablation of the His bundle for the treatment of medically refractory AV node re-entry tachycardia because it does not require a formal cardiac surgical operation. However permanent pacemaking systems are still required and the His catheter ablation technique is not without complications.

Because both His bundle cryoablation and His catheter ablation require permanent pacemaker systems a new technique was developed for the treatment of AV node reentry in which discrete cryo-surgical lesions are created around the borders of the AV node in an effort to alter the functional characteristics of the AV node while preserving atrioventricular conduction. In performing the discreet cryosurgical procedure, as many as nine separate 3- mm. cryolesions are placed around the borders of the triangle of Koch. The discreet cryolesions are applied until either a temporary block of AV conduction or permanent prolongation of the A-H interval occurs, at which time the cryothermic application is discontinued. In experimental studies those animals experiencing complete AV block exhibited a return of AV conduction with a prolonged A-H interval within 3 hours following cryothermic application. Three animals were found to have dual AV node conduction pathways considered to be the electrophysiologic substrate of AV node reeptry tachycardia. In all three, the discreet cryosurgical technique was capable of ablating one of the two AV node pathways, thus removing the anatomic-electrophysiologic substrate believed to be responsible for AV node reentry tachycardia. In four patients the dual AV node conduction pathways have been altered so that postoperatively only a single smooth AV node pathway exists with normal AV conduction and no further AV node reentry tachycardia has occurred.

Ectopic (Automatic) Atrial Tachycardia

Several patients with severe recurrent supraventricular tachycardia shown by electrophysiologic studies to be based on an ectopic (automatic) focus in the left atrium. These patients were unresponsive to all efforts of medical treatment. Since the preoperative electrophysiologic studies documented the site of ectopic activity to be in the left atrium, an attempt was made to localize precisely the site of ectopic activity by intraoperative electrophysiologic studies so that local surgical ablation of the ectopic focus could be performed. Unfortunately, due to the fact that arrhythmias occurring as a result of automatic activity are unresponsive to standard programmed electrical stimulation techniques as opposed to those resulting from a reentry mechanism, it may not be possible to map the supraventricular tachycardia during the surgical procedure. As a result these patients have all required surgical ablation of the bundle of His with insertion of a permanent ventricular pacemaker. Though this technique prevents the ventricles from responding to the supraventricular tachycardia, the undesirable side effect of this procedure is a lifelong dependence on an artificial ventricular pacing system. Since the ages of these patients have ranged from 16 to 32 years efforts were made to develop a surgical technique that would not require a permanent pacemaker. A procedure was developed in the laboratory which was really left atrial isolation so that the left atrium activity was isolated from the remaining heart. This allows the remaining heart to continue in a normal sinus rhythm This precludes the necessity for an artificial pacing system.

Atrial Flutter/Fibrillation Chronic atrial/flutter is present in approximately 60% of all patients undergoing isolated mitral valve replacement. Although there is no conclusive evidence that these arrhythmias originate preferentially in the left atrium in patients with mitral valve disease it appears reasonable to assume that in patients with left atrial hypertrophy and a normal right atrium atrial flutter/fibrillation most likely originates in the hypertrophied left atrial muscle. Because the left atrial isolation procedure is also capable of confining fibrillation to the left atrium this procedure is now being evaluated to determine its capability of alleviating the detrimental postoperative effects of atrial fibrillation in patients undergoing surgery for mitral valve replacement. Paroxysmal atrial flutter/fibrillation and chronic atrial/ flutter fibrillation are occasionally refractory to all medical therapy and the ventricular response rate during the arrhythmia may not be controlled by digoxin. In such instances the technique described above for discrete cryosurgery around the borders of the AV node may be capable of controlling the ventricular response rate to atrial flutter/ffibrillation. It is possible to induce permanent prolongation of the A-H interval in experimental studies without causing complete heart block using the discreet cryosurgery technique. In addition incremental atrial pacing and programmed electrical stimulation of the atrium have shown permanent alteration in the functional refractory period of the AV node and of the atrial pacing cycle length at which Wenckebach periodicity first occurs. By inducing these changes in AV node function the discrete cryosurgical technique can decrease permanently the ventricular response rate to supraventricular tachycardia in animals.

Postoperative Supraventricular Arrhythmias

Since the introduction of cold potassium cardioplegic solutions for myocardial preservation, there has been an increase in the incidence of cardiac conduction abnormalities and arrhythmias in the immediate and early postoperative period. Before cold potassium cardioplegia was used widely for myocardial preservation during cardiac operations, the incidence of postoperative cardiac conduction defects was reported to be as low as 12% after valve operations and 4% after aorto-coronary by pass procedures. In more recent reports in which cold potassium cardioplegia was used for myocardial preservation the incidence of postoperative cardiac arrhythmias was 72 to 80% after valve operations and 44-60% after aorto-coronary bypass procedures.

These undesirable sequelae of cold cardioplegic arrest have been attributed to the known electrophysiologic effects of high potassium levels on specialized cardiac conduction tissues and the myocardium. However several arrythmogenic factors other than elevated potassium are unique to the use of metabolic, hypothermic arrest and may play an equally important role in the genesis of postoperative cardiac arrhythmias. Prolonged continuous periods during which the aorta is cross-clamped and no coronary blood flow is present may lead to varying degrees of of temporary or permanent myocardial ischemic injury regardless of the level of potassium in the tissue. These undesirable sequelae of cold cardioplegic arrest have been attributed generally to the known electrophysiologic effects of high potassium levels on specialized conduction cardiac tissues and the myocardium. However several arrythmogenic factors other than the elevated potassium are unique to the use of metabolic hypothermic arrest and may play an equally important role in the genesis of postoperative cardiac arrhythmias. Prolonged continuous periods during which the aorta is cross-clamped and no coronary blood flow is present may lead to varying degrees of temporary or permanent myocardial ischemic injury regardless of the level of potassium present in the tissue. Differential cooling of the heart in which the atrium is warmer than the ventricle may result in resumption of atrial activity during the aortic cross clamp period. This may lead to ischemia of the AV node resulting in postoperative conduction disturbances and reentrant supraventricular arrhythmias. As in any cardiac tissue the reversibility of these conduction disturbances is related inversely to the degree of ischemic injury. And to the relative sensitivity of the tissues to ischemia. The proximal portions of the His -Purkinje system (the His bundle and major bundle branches) are more sensitive to ischemic injury than are the more peripheral portions (the parietal purkinje network). This differential sensitivity to ischemic injury may explain why the AV node and proximal portions of the His-Pukinje systems are the regions in which post cardioplegic conduction disturbances occur most often. Experience in patients under going coronary bypass grafting, a marked disparity was noted in the ability to cool the atrial septum and ventricular septum. More-over atrial septal temperature returned to the temperature of the systemic perfusate (28degrees C) within 3 minutes following cessation of cardioplegic infusion whereas ventricular septal temperature remained at 15-20 degrees C. The effects of intermittent topical iced saline slush on atrial septal temperature was transient. Following the period of cardioplegic arrest (avg 29 minutes) patients demonstrated first degree atrioventricular block and the prolonged AV conduction persisted for at least 2 hours after release of the aortic clamp. The prolongation of AV conduction following cardioplegic arrest was verified in animals. Electrograms recorded from the atrial septum, the His bundle, and the ventricles documented that the AV interval was prolonged following cardioplegic arrest. By utilizing these multiple electrode recordings, the conduction delays were seen to be confined primarily to the AVnode region indicating that inadequate cardioplegic preservation of the atria and atrial septum was most likely responsible for the conduction delay that was documented following cardioplegic arrest both experimentaly and clinically. Augmented cooling of the atria and the atrial septum prevented the post cardioplegic arrest conduction abnormalities. Thus it is obviously important to maintain adequate atrial hypothermia during the period of cardioplegic arrest to decrease the likelihood of postoperative conduction defects and supra-ventricular arrhythmias.

Ventricular Tachyarrythmias

Among the most common and lethal of arrhythmias are those arising in the ventricles. Although the medical treatment of ventricular arrhythmias particularly those associated with ischemic heart disease has improved in the past decade, a group of patients remains in whom ventricular arrhythmias are refractory to medical treatment. The term ventricular arrhythmias is usually associated with ischemic heart disease, but there are many kinds of ventricular arrhythmias unrelated to coronary heart disease. Most of the ventricular arrhythmias unassociated with coronary heart disease are remarkably intractable to medical therapy. As a result there has been increased emphasis on the surgical therapy of these arrhythmias.

Ventricular Tachyarrythmias Unrelated to Ischemic Heart Disease

Idiopathic ventricular tachycardia refers to patients in whom the only clinical manifestation of cardiac disease is the arrhythmia. Both the macroscopic appearance of the heart at operation and the pathologic data acquired at the time of autopsy in such patients fail to show any evidence of primary cardiac disease. The only abnormality noted has been global dilatation of the heart due to functional post-tachycardia heart failure. If these patients require surgery they first undergo intraoperative electrophysiological mapping during ventricular tachycardia in an effort to localize the origin of the arrhythmia. Surgical procedures have included simple ventriculotomy, exclusion procedures, and cryoablation. However the results have been poor because many of these arrhythmias arise within the ventricular septum. A small group of patients have been shown to have ventricular tachycardia due to non-ischemic cardiomyopathy. In this group angiographic and catheter data indicate some type of abnormal myocardial contractility associated with recurrent ventricular tachycardia. These patients usually show a diffuse dilatation of both ventricles with widespread patchy myocardial fibrosis. These tachyarrythmias frequently arise in the right ventricle and one approach to such patients has been to use a combination of surgical isolation and cryoablation of the origin of the arrhythmia. One patient, a 16 year old female with coxsackie B5 myocarditis, had intermittent ventricular tachycardia for 7 years following her initial viral infection. Preoperative electrophysiologic studies indicated that the ventricular tachycardia was arising from the pulmonary infundibulum near the level of the pulmonary valve annulus. However, the intraoperative studies showed that the tachycardia arose in the high right ventricular septum between the crista supraventricularis and the pulmonic valve annulus. A combination of surgical isolation and cryoablation of the origin of the ventricular tachycardia resulted in cessation of the arrhythmia. The patient remained free of ventricular tachycardia for 6 years and required no antiarrythmic drugs. Fontaine first described a previously unrecognized form of myopathy localized to the right ventricle to which he applied the term Arrythmogenic Right Ventricular Dysplasia. This syndrome appears to be a congenital cardiomyopathy characterized by transmuscular infiltration of adipose tissue resulting in weakness and bulging of the infundibulum, apex, and / or posterior basilar region of the right ventricle. The syndrome is characterized clinically by intractable ventricular tachycardia originating from one or all of the three pathologic areas of the right ventricle. Since the tachycardia is right ventricular in origin the standard ECG shows a pattern consistent with LBBB during the tachycardia. Right ventricular angiography should be performed in all patients who exhibit ventricular tachycardia with a LBBB pattern. In patients with arrythmogenic right ventricular dysplasia the right ventricle appears enlarged, ventricular bulges or frank aneurysms are seen in the infundibulum, the apex, and/ or the basal portion of the inferior wall. And right ventricular contractility is usually markedly decreased. Hypertrophic muscular bands in the infundibulum and anterior right ventricular wall result in apparent pseudodiverticula, leading to the so-called feathering appearance of the right ventricuiar outflow tract on angiography. Guiraudon has used simple ventriculotomies, aneurysm excision, or a combination of ventriculotomy and excision in 12 patients with one operative death and a 25% recurrence of ventricular tachycardia postoperatively. One approach to such patients was to use a transmural encircling ventriculotomy to isolated the arrythmogenic myocardium from the remainder of the heart. One patient was a 69 year old male with arrythmogenic right ventricular dysplasia in continuous ventricular tachycardia for 28 days prior to his operation. Preoperative electrophysiologic studies revealed the tachycardia to be originating from the posterior basilar region of the right ventricle. Intaoperative electrophysiologic studies revealed the tachycardia to be arising in the posterior- basilar region of the right ventricle adjacent to an area on the anterior right ventricle measuring 2×3cm that was electrically silent. In such cases one must recognize the possibility that the actual site of origin of the ventricular tachycardia may be in the electrically silent region It would appear to arise from the border of the silent region only because a certain critical mass of synchronously depolarized myocardium is essential to produce an ECG large enough to be detected by the exploring electrode. Since the three pathologically abnormal regions of the right ventricular dysplasia may exhibit electrical silence on epicardial mapping, every attempt should be made to isolate the entire pathologic area giving rise to the tachycardia from the remainder of the heart. The incision is begun in the atrioventricular groove at the level of the tricuspid valve annulus and is carried around the arrhythmogenic region of myocardium and returned to the level of the tricuspid annulus interiorly. At either end of the incision, a cryolesion is placed to ensure complete separation of all ventricular myocardial fibers on either side of the incision. A separate incision may be needed if there is a significant RV aneurysm. This patient remained free of ventricular arrhythmias for 5 years following surgery without antiarrhythmic drugs and and was hemodynamically normal. Intraoperative mapping of these patients has suggested that the entire right ventricle free-wall may be arrhythmogenic in certain cases. As a result our more recent approach to this problem has been to disconnect the entire right ventricular freewall from the remainder of the heart. The right ventricular disconnection procedure represents a logical extension of the two more localized right ventricular isolation procedures. The surgical technique for total right ventricular disconnection begins with a longitudinal ventriculotomy in the anterior right ventricle parallel to the interventricular septum approximately 5 mm to the right of the septum. This ventriculotomy is extended toward the apex and several trabeculae, including the moderator band of the right ventricle are transected sharply. The incision is then carried up to the pulmonary outflow tract just to the right of the interventricular septum to a point approximately 1mm across the anterior pulmonic valve annulus. A cryolesion is placed at the end of the incision across the pulmonic valve annulus The incision is then carried around the apex of the right ventricle Just to the right of the interventicular septum onto the posterior surface of the right ventricle. The posterior portion of the incision is extended to a point near the base of the heart approximately 1cm from the posterior tricuspid valve annulus. The remaining portion of the posterior incision is made from the endocardial aspect, but it continues to be transmural to the level of the posterior tricuspid valve annulus sparing only the AV groove pad and its encompassed coronary vessels. A cryolesion is placed at the distal end of the incision at the level of the posterior tricuspid valve annulus. Attention is directed to the supracristal ventricular septum between the posterior pulmonic valve annulus and the anterior medial tricuspid valve annulus. The His bundle and the right bundle branch are identified with a hand held electrode and an incision is placed between the posterior pulmonic valve annulus and the anterior medial tricuspid valve annulus from the endocardial aspect. The incision is transmural so that the aorta is visualized through the incision A cryolesion is placed at the end of the incision at the levels of the pulmonic valve annulus and the tricuspid valve annulus. The anterior papillary muscle is then transected at its base and reimplanted with multiple 3-0 pledgeted non-absorbable sutures onto the right ventricular septum. The entire right ventricular freewall is thus disconnected from the remainder of the heart except for the papillary muscle attachments to the posterior and septal leaflets of the tricuspid valve and these are attached to the right ventricular septum. Several cryolesions are placed at the base of these papillary muscles, preventing any possible electrical conduction from the papillary muscles to the right ventricle. The septal ventriculotomy between the posterior pulmonic valve annulus and the anterior medial tricuspid valve annulus is then closed with a continuous 3-0 non-absorbable suture. The long right free-wall ventriculotomy, which extends from the anterior pulmonic valve annulus down the anterior of the right ventricle, around the right ventricular apex and up the inferior right ventricular free-wall to the posterior tricuspid valve annulus, is closed with a single layer of 3-0 non-absorbable suture. This procedure isolates ventricular dysplasia from the remaining portion of the heart, allowing the heart to remain in normal sinus rhythm. We have now performed the right ventricular disconnection procedure successfully. Although the early results of the right ventricular disconnection procedure have been encouraging, a 3year followup in these patients indicates that a progressive dilatation of the right ventricle occurs to such an extent that overall left ventricular function may be compromised because of displacement of the ventricular septum. Although the potentially progressive nature of this problem remains unexplained it should be emphasized that that localized isolation procedures of the right ventricular free-wall should be done when possible and that total right ventricular disconnection procedure should be reserved for only the most serious and complex right ventricular tachyarrythmias.

Uhl's syndrome is a rare congenital cardiomyopathy that may be considered to be a more complete form of arrhythmogenic right ventricular dysplasia. The right ventricle is extremely dilated. The tricuspid valve remains in a normal position, differentiating it from Ebstein's anomaly. The main characteristic of Uhl's syndrome is the complete absence of myocardium in the right ventricular free wall, resulting in the endocardial and epicardial layers being indirect contact without interposition of myocardial fibers. Since Uhl's report of this cardiomyopathy in 1952 the descriptive term "parchment heart" has been applied to this abnormality. Although Uhl's syndrome usually leads to rapid cardiac failure in the first months or years of life, an adult form of the condition occurs in which associated ventricular tachycardia is the dominant feature. Although no surgical reatment has been applied for ventricular tachycardia associated with Uhl's syndrome, the development of the total right ventricular disconnection procedure promises to be of value in this unusual clinical problem.

In 1957, Jervell and Lange-Nielson described a clinical entity consisting of a long Q-T interval, congenital deafness, and syncopal attacks due to ventricular fibrillation following emotional or physical stresses. The absence of congenital deafness characterizes the identical Romano-ward syndrome. The Q-T interval prolongation in both these syndromes has been considered to be congenital in origen and both are recognized to contribute to sudden death in children. However in 1978, Schwartz demonstrated that certain patients who sustained acute myocardial infarctions subsequently developed Q-T interval prolongation and thereafter experienced a significantly higher incidence of sudden death. Although the pathogenesis of the long Q-T syndrome is poorly understood, James showed the presence of focal neuritis and neurodegeneration within the specialized conduction system and the ventricular myocardium. He suggested the possibility that a chronic viral infection or some non-infectious degeneration of the cardiac nerves might be responsible for the Q-T interval prolongation and for the associated fatal ventricular arrhythmias. Ventricular tachycardia that occurs in association with the long Q-T syndrome is frequently called torsade de pointes'. This term derives from the appearance of the ventricular tachycardia on a standard ECG in which the polarity of the tachycardia is inconstant. The electrcardiographic features of Torsade de pointes' are unique and may be described as follows: the episodes are generaly initiated by a ventricular ectopic beat following late after the preceding sinus complex (2) the successive QRS complexes during tachycardia show an undulating series of rotations of the electrical axis the episodes frequently cease spontaneously. In addition the arrhythmia is usually preceded by variations in the T wave during the last several beats prior to the development of the tachycardia. One of the most frequent causes of Torsade de pointes is the administration of medications particularly quinidine which prolong ventricular repolarization. These observations support the concept that torsade de pointes represents an abnormality in the myocardial repolarization. As a result the surgical treatment of recurrent ventricular tachycardia associated with the long Q-T syndrome has centered around efforts at modifying cardiac enervation. Yanowitz showed that unilateral alterations in sympathetic tone altered not only the shape of the T wave but also its duration (Q-T interval). His studies in animals showed that right stellate ganglion stimulation resulted in prolonged Q-T interval and increased T wave amplitude. Conversely, left stellate ganglion resection or right stellate ganglion stimulation produced increased T-wave negativity without measurable changes in the Q-T interval. These findings and those of others have led to the hypothesis that electrocardiographic changes following unilateral alterations of sympathetic tone provide a functional explanation for the electrocardiographic abnormalities seen in patients with lesions of the central nervous systemas well as with patients with the long Q-T syndrome. Left stellate ganglion resection has been reported to abolish symptoms in approximately 20 patients with the long Q-T syndrome. However experience with the left stellate ganglion resection for the treatment of 'torsate de pointes' associated with the long Q-T syndrome has been characterized by early success and late failure.

Ventricular Tachyarrythmias Associated With Ischemic Heart Disease

The common ventricular arrhythmias are those that occur in association with ischemic heart disease. Meticulous follow-up studies document that serious ventricular arrhythmias of this type are harbinger of sudden cardiac death within the first year after an acute myocardial infarction. Survival seems to be improved by antiarrhythmic drugs but the arrhythmias persist in many patients despite all combinations of pharmacologic therapy available. Many surgical techniques have been used in the past in an attempt to alleviate ventricular arrhythmias associated with coronary artery disease. It is necessary to understand the mechanisms of ventricular tachyarrhythmias associated with ischemic heart disease to decide whether or not surgery is indicated and to determine the optimal surgical approach. Cardiac rhythm reflects a balance or stable behavior resulting from a complex system of interacting anatomic and electrophysiologic variables. These components include normal or abnormal conduction pathways, homogeneous vs heterogeneous excitability, conduction, recovery, and exaggerated automaticity. Tachycardia represents an imbalance or unstable electrophysiologic state due to the interaction of these abnormal variables. Current concepts of the mechanisms of ventricular tachycardia associated with ischemic heart disease include re-entry, enhanced or abnormal automaticity, and triggered automaticity. Although the latter two mechanisms are believed to account for certain arrhythmias, reentry has been most convincingly documented in patients.

Older generalized concepts of the reentrant pathway were confined to relatively simple substrates of the Purkinje-myocardial junction models, when in fact they may be as complex as the heterogeneous three-dimensional structure of actual myocardial infarcts. Ischemic zones around myocardial infarctions have been described. Subsequent studies have modified the initial concept of this border zone but its importance in the genesis of ischemic ventricular tachyarrhythmias is well documented. Such studies in animal models and more recently in man suggest that most reentrant ventricular tachycardias in ischemic heart disease are primarily myocardial microentrant (confined to a relatively small area of contiguous myocardium) rather than microentrant (pathways involving broad Purkinje-myocardial loops) and more complex geometrically than previously thought. Reentrent ischemic ventricular arrhythmias result from complex interplay between (l) a non-uniform (hterogenous) state of repolarization (2) slow desynchronized conduction over. abnormal myocardial pathways created by fibrotic or ischemic discontinuity and (3) ventricular ectopy. Premature beats interacting with non-uniform (heterogenous) recovery result in regional differences in conduction of the impulse. Some regions fail to excite others excite but propagate slowly whereas immediately adjacent regions excite normally. The same impulse later invades regions not excited initially as they finally repolarize. Even later these delayed impulses reexcite or renter the areas first excited by the premature beat and are therefore first to repolarize. This type of reentry typically results in short cardiac cycles and fast rates I.E. ventricular fibrillation or flutter. Ventricular Tachycardia is determined by a longer reentrant cycle time that necessitates either complex dissociation and extreme slowing of the reentrant wave within a small area (microreentry) or circus like conduction over a long pathway (macroreentry). Slow, desynchronized conduction is a hallmark of myocardial injury or fibrosis. Conduction velocity depends on the synchrony of the activation process. Fibrosis is non-uniform at the borders of infarcts and produces complex interdigitations between normal myocardium and scar. Synchronous wavefronts, upon approaching such an area may become desynchronized, fragmenting into many individual wavelets. Slow conduction accompanies the desynchronization. Slow desynchronized conduction also can be produced by applying tension or compression forces to the myocardium. Tension forces existing at the margins of aneurysms or infarcts may extend or radiate through the myocardium resulting in desynchronization of activity or ectopy. This mechanism maybe similar to the myocardial compression reentry problem of Schmitt and Erlanger and probably explains why a standard left ventricular aneurysm resection occasionally results in relief of associated ventricular tachycardia. Since resection of the aneurysm alters overall left ventricular geometry, it would also be expected to alter the tension forces existing at the margin of the aneurysm and radiating through the adjacent myocardium. Whether these mechanical forces act through the induction of ischemia or act directly is unknown.

Preoperative Electrphysiologic Evaluation

The objectives of preoperative endocardial catheter mapping procedures are (1) confirmation that the arrhythmia is ventricular rather than supra ventricular in origin, (2) demonstration that the ventricular arrhythmia can be induced and terminated by programmed electrical stimulation techniques i.e. that it is a reentrant arrhythmia, and (3) localization of the region of origin or ventricular tachycardia when possible. This study usually demonstrates the arrhythmia to be ventricular tachycardia of a single morphologic type, indicating that it is originating from a single region in the left ventricle. Following induction these monomorphic ventricular tachycardias are usually sustained for a sufficient length of time to allow endocardial catheter mapping to determine their site of origin. However monomorphic ventricular tachycardia may be nonsustained, thus precluding adequate mapping during the preoperative electrophysiology study. The preoperative study may also document the arrhythmia to be Polymorphic Ventricular Tachycardia. This term is applied not only to ventricular tachycardia that originates from several different regions of the left ventricle giving rise to several different morphologic types of tachycardia but also tachycardia that originates from one general region of the left ventricle but is characterized electrophysiologically by excessive fragmentation such that individual depolarization complexes may be difficult to identify. Polymorphic ventricular tachycardia may also be sustained or nonsustained but it commonly deteriorates rather quickly into ventricular fibrillation. Electrophysiologic deterioration to ventricular fibrillation may be the result of primary electrical instability or it may occur because of hemodynamic compromise associated with the onset of polymorphic ventricular tachycardia. The third type of refractory ischemic ventricular tachyarrhythmia is Primary Ventricular Fibrillation which is identified during the preoperative electrophysiology by the absence of any type of induced ventricular tachycardia prior to the onset of ventricular fibrillation.

Surgical Indications and Contraindications

Major indications for surgical intervention in ischemic ventricular tachyarrhythmias include medical refractoriness to ventricular tachycardia, patient intolerance to effective medical treatment and poor patient compliance. A specific surgical procedure directed at the arrhythmiais also indicated in patients with intractable angina pectoris requiring coronary artery bypass grafting who have associated ventricular tachycardia and in patients with congestive heart failure due to a left ventricular aneurysm requiring resection who have associated ventricular tachycardia. The contraindications to surgical intervention for ischemic tachyarrhythmias are determined by the preoperative electrophysiology study and include noninducible ventricular tachycardia, and non-sustained polymorphic ventricular tachycardia.

Following an electrophysiolgic study, surgery is usually not feasible since the induction of the arrhythmia intraoperatively would be extremely unlikely. Likewise if the patient is found to have nonsustained polymorphic ventricular tachycardia during the preoperative electrophysiology study, it is highly unlikely that the arrhythmia could be induced intraoperatively long enough to identify its site of origin. However if the nonsustained polymorphic ventricular tachycardia has proved to be life threatening, one of the non-localized direct endocardial surgical procedures that does not require intraoperative elctrophysiologic mapping may be indicated as a last resort. As mentioned previously the surgical results of treatment of automatic ventricular tachyarrhythmias has been notoriously unsuccessful. Likewise there is, no surgical procedure available for the prevention of primary ventricular fibrillation. But it can be treated by an automatic internal defibrillator.

Intraoperative Mapping Procedure

The primary objective of intraoperative electrophysiologic mapping is to localize the arrhythmogenic region of the left ventricle that gives rise to ventricular tachycardia. Localization of the origin of the tachycardia guides the surgeon in determining the appropriate type of operative procedure and the region to which it should be applied. Since the majority of refractory ischemic ventricular tachyarrhythmias are generated from microreentrant circuits, the apparent site of arrhythmogenesis is usually comfined to a small area of the left ventricular septum or free-wall. Epicardial intramural and endocardial isosynchronous electrophysiologic maps are constructed during normal sinus rhythm and during induced ventricular tachycardia. The normal sinus rhythm maps are performed to identify areas where simple or complex fragmentation of the local electrogram occurs, indicating the regions that are most likely to harbor latent microentrant circuits. Programmed electric stimulation or burst pacing of the ventricle is then performed to induce ventricular tachycardia.

Several factors make it more difficult to induce ventricular tachycardia intraoperatively than preoperatively. These factors include general anesthesia, decreased myocardial temperature because of intraoperative cardiac exposure, subtle changes in left ventricular geometry, and wall tension and cardiac manipulation during cannulation for cardio-pulmonary bypass. However, ventricular tachycardia sustained long enough to allow adequate intraoperative mapping can be induced in most patients. All antiarrhythmic medications should be discontinued 24 hours preoperatively, if possible, and their use should should be avoided during anesthetic induction. Intracardiac monitoring catheters e.g. Swan-Gantz catheters are not used preoperatively, and gentle handling of the heart during cannulation and during normal sinus rhythm mapping is mandatory. The institution of cardiopulmonary bypass provides a safe means of altering left ventricular preload and thus wall tension, and thus permits control of myocardial temperature. Elevation of myocardial temperature between 38 and 38.5 degrees C is frequently helpful in providing the necessary milieu for induction of sustained ventricular tachycardia. In addition the use of pulsatile cardiopulmonary bypass may increase the ability to sustain stable ventricular tachycardia intraoperatively.

Because of the frequent inability to induce ventricular tachycardia that is sustained long enough to allow complete mapping, several investigators have worked on developing a computerized system that will allow the ventricles to be mapped from a short run of nonsustained or polymorphic ventricular tachycardia. Such a system has now been developed by Witkowski and Corr at Washigton University Medical Center, Barnes Hospital in St Louis and it is used routinely by a number of cardiac surgical teams for the intraoperative activation sequences In patients undergoing surgery for tachyarrhythmias as well as for surgery for WPW syndrome. Multiple transmural 22 gauge needle electrodes with contact points every mm along the needle shaft are inserted through the left ventricular and/ or right ventricular freewall and septum, and transmural isochronous maps are constructed during normal sinus rhythm. Programmed electrical stimulation or burst pacing techniques are the used to induce ventricular tachycardia and transmural maps are again constructed to determine the earliest site of activity during the tachycardia. The electrograms are filtered and digitized in individual specially designed amplifiers and the digitized data are relayed via a fiberoptic cable for processing. A computer generated, multicolored, isochronous map is then displayed in the operating room 120 seconds later. Maps for any level of the myocardial wall from endocardium to epicardium can be visualized, thus providing precise localization of the site of origin of the ventricular tachycardia. Earliest endocardial activity most commonly occurs before earliest epicardial activity. But intramural activity frequently occurs before endocardial activation. The latter observation confirms that many microentrant circuits responsible for refractory ischemic ventricular tachycardia are located intramurally and not in the subendocardium or endocardium. The microentrant circuits still may arise from the border zone junction between fibrosis and normal myocardium since this zone is not confined to the endocardium. Although the earliest activity during ventricular tachycardia may occur intramurally the subjacent endocardium is usually activated before the overlying epicardium. This observation may indicate that the intramural reentrant circuit is located closer to the endocardium, or it may reflect a more rapid conduction of electrical activity through endocardial Purkinje fibers that have survived the previous myocardial infarction.

Surgical Procedures

In a recent review of the literature, 171 patients were reported to have one of four different types of indirect surgical procedures for the treatment of recurrent ventricular arrhythmias associated with coronary artery disease. Thoracic sympathectomy, coronary artery bypass grafting, heart wall resection, or a combination of coronary bypass grafting and resection was used in these patients with an overall operative mortality of 27%, a failure rate of 17%, and an overall success rate of 56%. Because of the unsatisfactory results obtained with these indirect procedures, direct endocardal approaches guided by intraoperative electrophysiologic mapping procedures were introduced. Direct surgical procedures may be classified as ablation or isolation operations. Surgical isolation procedures are designed not to ablate the arrhythmia per se but rather to confine it to a specific region of the heart. Ablative surgical procedures are of two types: those that interrupt one limb of a reentrant circuit and those that destroy or remove the anatomic substrate harboring a reentrant circuit or automatic focus. The first direct endocardial procedure specifically developed for the treatment of ventricular tachycardia associated with ischemic heart disease was the encircling endocardial ventriculotomy (EEV) described by Guiraudon in 1978. He reasoned that since ventricular tachycardia associated with previous myocardial infarctions arose as a result of reentrant circuits in the border zone, a standard left ventricular aneurysmectomy that leaves this border zone intact should not be expected to ablate the arrhythmia with any degree of regularity. In his procedure an endocardial incision is placed just outside the juncture of endocardial fibrosis and normal endocardium and is carried around the entire base of the aneurysm or infarction. The incision is essentially transmural sparing only the overlying epicardial vessels and a superficial bridge of subepicardial muscle on the free wall, It is placed one cm deep in the septum. Guiraudon initially proposed the operation as an isolation procedure and it may function as such in some instances. However experimental studies have shown that its most common mechanism of action is ablative, since the EEV causes a marked decrease in myocardial blood flow to the encompassed myocardium when applied to anterior left ventricular aneurysms. The decreased regional myocardial blood flow is believed to result in ablation of the anatomic- electrphysiologic substrate responsible for the arrhythmia by disrupting the delicate imbalance necessary for perpetuation of a microreentrant tachyarrhythmia. One side effect of using an EEV in anterior aneurysms is a decrease in regional function of the encompassed myocardium that may aggravate the low output syndrome in patients with large left ventricular aneurysms. The most widely used procedure for the treatment of refractory ischemic ventricular tachycardia is the localized endocardial resection procedure (ERP) first described by Josepheson, Horowitz, and Harken. This procedure is clearly an ablative one in which the arrhythmogenic region identified by endocardial mapping is excised. The concept that this region is confined to the endocardium is erroneous since the junction between fibrosis and normal myocardium extends from the endocardium to the epicardium in transmural infarcts and aneurysms., However since this junction is also the location of the border zone that gives rise to reentrant ventricular tachycardia and since it is destroyed by removing the fibrosis, the endocardial resection procedure has been quite effective in ablating refractory ischemic ventricular tachycardia. Its success is dependant on the correct identification of the arrythmogenic locale around the circumference of the aneurysm base, as defined by the site of earliest endocardial activation during ventricular tachycardia. It does not require determination of the exact site of origin of the ventricular tachycardia in relation to its intramural depth. Thus, a given arrhythmia could originate from a micro-entrant circuit located in the mid-myocardium at the junction of fibrotic and normal myocardium and propagate to both the epicardium and endocardium arriving at the endocardium earlier because of surviving Purkinje fibers. The endocardial isochronous map would demonstrate a site of earliest activation and the endocardial fibrosis in that region of the aneurysm would be resected. As the dissection progressed from endocardium to epicardium in that region, the mid-myocardial reentant circuit would be excised and the ventricular tachycardia would be ablated. Thus, the fact that intramural studies have documented many cases of refractory ischemic ventricular tachycardia originating in the mid-myocardium does not detract from the usefulness or effectiveness of the ERP provided the border zone is disrupted or excised when the fibrosis is removed. The major disadvantage of the ERP is that it cannot be applied safely for the treatment of arrhythmias arising from the papillary muscles or from regions near the aortic or mitral valve annulus. Another disadvantage is that stable ventricular tachycardia frequently is not sustained long enough intraoperatively to allow accurate electrophysiologic localization of the site of origin unless a computerized mapping system is available to the surgeon. Ventricular tachycardias of multiple morphologic types arising from several different areas within the left ventricle may require more extensive endocardial resection., Primarily because of the latter problem, Moran modified the localized endocardial resection procedure to include resection of all the fibrosis associated with with a left ventricular aneurysm or infarction, an approach termed the "extended" endocardial resection procedure (EERP). This operation has been shown to be extremely effective in controlling refractory ischemic ventricular tachyarrhythmias unless they arise from the papillary muscles or in regions adjacent to the aortic or mitral valve annulus. In those instance, the EERP suffers from the same limitations in application as does the localized ERP. Finally endocardial ablation was introduced as both a primary form of therapy and as an adjunctive procedure to be employed with an EEV, ERP or EERP. A 1.5 cm diameter cryoprobe, cooled with internally expanding nitrous oxide to -60 degrees C is placed over the site of earliest endocardial activity during ventricular tachycardia. Permanent cryoablation is attained after 2 minutes of application. The advantage of cryosurgery over the other techniques are its versatility and preciseness, Its rapid application and the fact that cryothermia is the only ablative procedure that preserves tissue collagen and thus ventricular wall integrity. Moreover cryosurgery may be applied safely to any endocardial surface within the heart except for regions near the bundle of His, where it may cause permanent atrioventricular conduction block.

EEV (encircling endocardial ventriculotomy)
WPW (Wolff Parkinson White)
LBBB (left bundle branch block)
RBBB (right bundle branch block
SA (sinoatrial node)
AV (atrioventricular node)
PSVT (paroxysmal supraventricular tachycardia)

Arrythmogenic right ventricular dysplasia (congenital cardiomyopathy with transmural infiltration of adipose tissue resulting in weakness and bulging of the infundibulum, apex, and/or posterior-basilar region of the right ventrical)

EERP (extended endocardial resection procedure)
EEV (Encircling endocardial ventriculotomy)
ERP (endocardial resection procedure)

Current Procedures of Choice for Refactory Ischemic Ventricular Tachycardia

The surgical approach in a given patient with refractory ischemic ventricular atachycardia should depend on two factors (1) The electrophysiologic characteristics of the ventricular tachycardia and (2) the anatomic site of origin of the ventricular tachycardia. Sustained monomorphic ventricular tachycardia can be mapped easily intraoperatively and its site of origin can be identified without difficulty. Proper localization of the site of origin of nonsustained monomorphic ventricular tachycardia may be very difficult intraoperatively unless an electrophysiologic mapping system capable of recording multiple electrograms simultaneously is available. In general these types of arrhythmias must be treated with a less localized procedure than those employed for tachycardias that are sustained long enough for accurate intraoperative localization of the arrhythmogenic site. Likewise polymorphic ventricular tachycardia routinely requires one of the less localized procedures.

Ventricular Tachycardia Arising from the Anterior or Lateral Left Ventricle

If the anterior left ventricular septum is found to be the arrhythmogenic site and the tachycardia is sustained and monomorphic the localized endocardial resection procedures should be employed. If the tachycardia cannot be mapped sufficiently because it is nonsustained, an extended ERP (extended resection) should be performed to avoid the likelihood of recurrence postoperatively. If the tachycardia arising in this region is polymorphic it may be necessary to resect all of the endocardial fibrosis associated with the left ventricular aneurysm. (EERP) (extended endocardial resection procedure) but also to perform endocardial cryoablation in the area that shows the greatest fragmentation during normal sinus rhythm mapping., Tachycardias arising in the lateral free-wall are approached in the same manner. If the anterior papillary muscle can be demonstrated to be the arrhythmogenic site of either a sustained or non-sustained monomorphic tachycardia, endocardial cryoablation of the lower two thirds of the papillary muscle should be performed. If the tachycardia appears to be arising from the anterior papillary, but is polymorphic, all of the endocardial fibrosis associated with the aneurysm should be resected and endocardial ablation should be applied to the lower 2/3 of the papillary muscle.

Ventricular Tachyarrythmias Arising in the Posterior Left Ventricle
Ventricular tachyarrhythmias arising in the posterior region of the left ventricle are more difficult to treat surgically because of two technical problems. The involves the difficulty in mapping these patients even with a sustained ventricular tachycardia because of the necessity, to retract the ventricular apex out of the pericardial sac. A longitudinal left ventriculotomy must be placed between the base of the posterior papillary muscle and the posterior interventricular septum and the posterior endocardium must then be mapped through this posterior

ventriculotomy. Such retraction of the heart frequently induces significant aortic insufficiency, which may preclude ones ability to identify accurately the site of origin of the arrhythmia. The second technical problem in this region involves the potential disruption of either the aortic or mitral valve apparatus by the surgical procedure itself. Experience has shown that these tachyarrhythmias usually originate extremely close to the junction of the aortic and mitral valves and that resection of the endocardial fibrosis to within 3 to 5 mm of the valve annuli frequently does not interrupt the tachycardia. These technical difficulties are magnified if the patient has only a posterior myocardial infarction rather than a posterior left ventricular aneurysm associated with the ventricular tachycardia. If the arrhythmogenic site of ventricular tachycardia can be localized to the posterior papillary muscle endocardial cryoablation of the papillary muscle should be performed. However, if the tachycardia is nonsustained so that one cannot be certain that the arrhythmogenic site is in the posterior papillary muscle an EEV may be placed around the entire border of fibrosis on the posterior papillary wall, papillary muscle, and posterior LV septum. The EEV (encircling endocardial ventriculotomy) incision is based medially on the aortic valve annulus and laterally on the mitral valve annulus and is carried to within 5 mm of each annulus. An endocardial cryolesion is placed at either end of the EEV incision to complete the "encirclement' of the fibrotic myocardium containing the base of posterior papillary muscle. The resultant 'pedicle' of left ventricular myocardium receives its blood supply from posterior lateral branches of the right or circumflex coronary arteries and thus neither regional myocardial blood flow nor regional myocardial function of the encircled myocardium should be affected by the incision. This is substantiated by the fact that no instances of mitral dysfunction have been reported following EEV's incorporating the papillary muscle within the incision.

Polymorphic ventricular tachycardia arising from the posterior left ventricular free-wall is managed in an identical manner. However, if the arrhythmogenic site can be localized accurately to the posterior free-wall it is preferable to performa localized endocardial resection procedure. In the case of non-sustained tachycardia arising from this region, either an extended ERP or an EEV may be performed as the primary procedure with endocardial cryoablation being applied near the aortic and/or mitral valve annulus. If tachycardia arising from the posterior left ventricular septum can be localized adequately one may perform a localized ERP, but cryoablation near the aortic annulus is usually indicated as well. If the tachycardia cannot be localized satisfactorily within the posterior septum or posterior papillary muscle because it is either non-sustained or polymorphic, It is preferable to resect all of the endocardial fibrosis (EERP) and apply endocardial cryolesions along the aortic and mitral valve, annuli and over the base of the posterior papillary muscle. It is apparent that the specific surgical procedure applied in a given patient with refractory ischemic ventricular tachycardia must be tailored to the anatomic and electrophysiologic characteristics presented by each individual case. It is extremely important to perform these surgical procedures during induced ventricular tachycardia when the arrhythmia is sustained or to perform the procedures in the beating non-working heart in the case of non-sustained ventricular tachycardia. Immediately, after performing the specific endocardial procedure they repeatedly attempt to reinduce the arrhythmia until they are convinced that it can no longer be induced., By performing the procedure without utilizing cardioplegic arrest the potential temporary salutary effects of hypothermia and of the cardioplegic solution itself are eliminated. It is felt that the 20% reinducibility rate of ventricular tachycardia during the postoperative electrphysiologic study in most reported series is related to the fact that these surgical procedures are commonly performed during cardioplegic arrest and that the temporary effects of hypothermia and/or cardioplegia result in a lack of inducibility in the operating room immediately following surgery despite the fact that the tachycardia can be induced 7 to 10 days later in one of every five patients. By employing the surgical procedures as outlined without employing cardioplegic arrest, we have had no postoperative recurrences of ventricular tachycardia, and only one patient had one of his four types of ventricular tachycardia induced at the time of his postoperative study.

In summary it has become possible to treat refractory ischemic ventricular tachycardia in a safe effective and predictable fashion. All of the direct endocardial surgical procedures are effective in a given situation and if applied in a logical manner based upon preoperative and intraoperative electrphysiologic data they are almost uniformly successful incontrolling these life- threatening tachyarrhythmias. Exercise or angina induced ventricular tachyarrhythmias are another subset of these patients and for the moment it is not recommended to have an extensive and risky operation for tachyarrythmias that occur only during angina or exercise. It is reasoned that some of these patients should undergo coronary angiography and bypass grafting of the appropriate coronary arteries.

CHAPTER 7

Perspectives Of Thoracic Surgery

THERE IS INCREASING awareness of the discrepancy between the pathologic findings and the presence of heart block. Fibrosis localized to the conduction bundle unrelated to vascular disease is a common finding. Rheumatic valvular disease found in 5% to 10% of the patients with complete or high grade heart block is almost always aortic valvular disease with calcific invasion of the adjacent septum. Penton et al reported the presence of heart block in 12 patients with mitral valve disease. Luetic heart disease, congenital defects, the residua of diphtheria, lupus erythematosus, sarcoidosis uremia, chagas disease, and familial cardiomyopathy are other causes. Digitalis intoxication may be a precipitating cause in the development of Stokes-Adams Disease in patients with atrial fibrillation and associated partial or complete heart block. Digitalis can depress impulse initiation, prevent conduction through the atrioventricular node, cause paroxysmal tachycardia and produce ventricular fibrillation. The reported incidence of temporary heart block in acute myocardial infarction is significant, as high as 25% in some series. Heart block arising in the acute phase of a myocardial infarction is significant, as high as 25% in some series. Heart block arising in the acute phase of a myocardial infarction rarely becomes a chronic problem requiring implantation of a pacemaker, the conduction defect disappears in one or two weeks. In these cases pathologic studies have revealed only minimal lesions of the conduction system. There may be a need for temporary artificial pacing in some patients and there may be a need for a permanent implantation of a battery run pacemaker in others. Statistics indicate that anterior myocardial infarction with aberrant types of QRS conduction is associated with a high mortality, the result of atrioventricular block. Heart block following operations for congenital or acquired heart disease is related to injury to the conduction system. This may be related to injury to the conduction system by suture, hemorrhrage or necrosis. Injury may result in evanescent, temporary or, complete heart block. Hemorrhages, some with necrosis as a result of a suture passing through the bundle, encircling the bundle or in the vicinity of the bundle and are most apt to occur following closure of ventricular septal defects. Refinements of suturing technique have reduced this to less than 1%. Complete heart block following replacement of the aortic valve have been frequent. In some series although half were of a transitory nature. Severe calcific aortic stenosis with calcification invading or penetrating the annulus is the common factor in these. Sutures placed at the lower most portion of the noncoronary cusp were found to penetrate the entire thickness of the of the atrial wall in the region of the bundle of his. Clinical course poses the danger of sudden death.

Heart failure, dyspnea and angina are related. Syncope is the result of transient reduction or sudden interruption of circulation. The convulsions of a true Stokes-Adams attack result from more prolonged episodes of asystole or the arrhythmias of ventricular fibrillation and ventricular tachycardia. They need to be differentiated from those of carotid vessel occlusion and intracerebral vascular disease. Carotid vessel occlusion and intracerebral disease are more likely to manifest unilateral blindness and muscle weakness rather than syncope as in bradycardia or asystole. Data on survival after the onset of complete heart block vary but Friedberg et al found that 50% of a group of 100 patients were dead within a year of onset. Lawrence et al in a review of 49 patients with complete heart block secondary to arteriosclerotic disease followed over a 20 year period found that the majority were in the sixth and seventh decades of life. Twenty per cent died suddenly. Nine patients lived with restriction of activity from nine to fourteen years after onset. Nearly all a had persistence of heart failure or hypertension. Obviously there was a pressing need to develop a means of pacing the heart both in cardiology in general especially in cardiac surgery as it developed. Development of the implantable pacemaker which has become a standard and sophisticated instrument has progressed from single wire electrodes advanced through an arm vein to the right ventricle from an external battery pack or electricle stimulater to implantable units connected to the heart usually the left ventricle directly from an implanted unit in the upper abdominal wall or an electrode to the right ventricle from a battery unit in the right upper chest wall. Both unipolar or bipolar catheter can be used. A variety of pacing modes are available, from asynchronous to synchronous to demand pacing when the rhythm is intermittent and unreliable. The most recent pacemakers will not only provide pacing in a synchronous fashion but will defibrillate the heart should asystole occur. These are marvelous bits of electronics and are a far cry from the original implanted pacemaker first used by Paul Zoll in 1952. Occasionally temporary wires attached to the right atrial appendage are used if there is a danger of heart block because of the technique or the location of the bundle or the proximity of the sutures. If some form of heart block occurs or there is a danger of developing heart block postop the patient can be paced and the pacing wire can be removed without having to enter the chest when the danger of heart block has passed. Atrioventricular synchronous pacers are available for those in whom the atrial contribution is important and for whom the atrium provides a means of adjusting ventricular rate to the to the requirements of stress. An atrioventricular sequential demand pacemaker consists of two stimulating catheters one atrial and one ventricular. Both stimulators are recycled by sensing a ventricular R wave. The atrial electrode only stimulates and the ventricular electrode serves as a sensor as well as a stimulater. The mechanism is such that the pacemaker may remain dormant or, may function as a preset pacer, or may stimulate both atria and ventricles in synchrony. Other designs allow sensing of the atrial impulse with a 390-msec delay to simulate a normal atrioventricular sequence. There are unipolar and bipolar catheters available. A bipolar catheter has both cathode and anode at the tip of the cathether approximately 1 cm apart. A large variety Of permanent pacemakers is available. Batteries have a different lifespan, the most recent one is the lithium iodide with functional lives of 10 to 20 years. I think it is safe to say that all these mechanical and electrical parts replacement represent gigantic advancements cardiac surgery as a science and a life saving modality.

CONCEPT IN PCI

Percutaneous coronary Intervention

Percutaneous coronary intervention. This is a technique of placing stents in the coronary arteries to solve problems of stenosis or complete obstruction of the coronary arteries as an emergency resulting from acute infarction or as an elective procedure in patients with symptomatic stenosis or obstruction. Stents either bare or drug eluting stents have been placed at the site of obstruction to relieve symptoms or as treatment in the case of myocardial infarction. The procedure is a percutaneous coronary intervention from either the femoral or radial arteries. Thus the designation of PCI or percutaneous coronary intervention. There has been an evolution in stent design as well as in the drugs they elute. The transcatheter approach also includes a consideration of the trans- catheter aortic valve replacement. Vascular injury and platelet activation after intracoronary implantation require systemic (DAPT) dual antiplatelet to lessen the risk for near-term thrombotic events. This course is extended in the setting of DES (drug eluting stents) because antiproliferative agents inhibit vascular healing and stent endothelialization. Randomized trials leading to regulatory approval of first generation paclitaxel-eluting and sirolimus- eluting stents which tended to enroll low-risk patients and /or lesions suggested that DAPT (dual anti-platelet)durations of 3- 6 months may be sufficient after implantation of paclitaxel- eluting and sirolimus -eluting stents, respectively. Subsequent analysis involving real world patients challenged this notion by demonstrating a higher thrombotic risk with the use of first –generation DES(drug eluting stents)versus bare-metal stents (BMS)particularly when implanted in an off label fashion. Moreover other reports suggested that sustained or prolonged DAPT(dual anti platelet therapy) may yield a protective benefit. Among patients treated with DES (drug- eluting stents)who were event free at either 6 or 12 months, Eisenstein et al found that clopidogrel use was associated with significant reductions in death and death or myocardial infarction at up to 24 months after PCI(Percutaneous coronary intervention). In contrast, no apparent advantage was observed for prolonged dopidogrel use among patients treated with BMS(

Bare metal stents). Analogously, Iakovou et al found that the premature discontinuation of (DAPT) dual anti-platelet therapy was the strongest predictor of stent thrombosis among patients receiving first generation drug eluting stents (DES). Among diabetic patients, Brar et al also found a protective effect of prolonged (DAPT) dual anti-platelet therapy. While much of the activity is placing drug eluting stents in patients with coronary occlusive disease there are a sizable number of patients who have been treated with saphenous vein bypass, a number of these show up later with stenosis or occlusion of the graft and automatically become candidates for PCI (percutaneous coronary intervention). Dept of Veterans Affairs Cooperative study showed a 10 year patency rate of SVGs at 61%. This is expected to become a more frequent problem as the patients with saphenous vein bypass age. In addition patients with coronary bypass procedures undergoing percutaneous coronary intervention(PCI) have a higher procedural- risk and in-hospital mortality than patients undergoing PCI (percutaneous coronary intervention)in native coronary arteries. Wojakowski and Wojiech Wanha in Concepts in PCI describe one such case using a self-expandable Stentys stent to avoid distal embolization and to optimize the apposition of the stent to the vessel wall. The stent has self expansion properties which over time prevents undersizing the stent and also facilitates containment of the thrombus between struts and vessel wall.

This is a very short introduction into the complexities of the PCI world. While we cannot strictly call it thoracic surgery it has become an important tool for the surgeon doing coronary artery bypass grafting.

CHAPTER 8

Chest Implanted LVAD

THE HEART WARE Ventricular Assist System, a small left ventricular assist device that is implanted in the chest instead of the abdomen has been approved by the Food and Drug Administration as a bridge to heart transplant for the end-stage heart failure patients. The Heartware Ventricular System includes an implantable pump with an external driver and power source. The device is another treatment option for advanced heart failure patients, especially those who are smaller in size or can't have an abdominal implant. The approval of the continuous flow pump device comes less than 3 years after the agency approved Thoratec's HeartMate II left ventricular assist device (LVAD) for destination therapy. That device quickly replaced the previous generation of pulsatile devices. This is the first time that the FDA has approved a ventricular assist device using comparator data from a registry as a control, according to the agency.

The approval was based on data from the ADVANCE trial, which compared the outcomes of 137 patients implanted with the HeartWare System and of patients registered by the Interagency Registry for Mechanically Assisted Circulatory Support (INTERMACS). The registry has been in place since 2005. A total of 140 patients received the investigational pump and 499 patients received a commercially available pump implanted contemporaneously. At 180 days, 90.7% of the investigational pump patients and 90.1% of the of the controls had survived establishing the non-inferiority of the investigational pump. Induction right heart failure, device replacement, stroke, kidney dysfunction, hemolysis, and arrhythmia rates for the HVAD were similar to those reported previously for the HeartMate II.

Results of the ADVANCE trial showed that at 6 months, median 6-minute walk distance were improved by 128.5 meters and functional capacity and quality of life improved markedly and the adverse event profile was favorable. HeartWare registry data facilitated the development and availability of this new device. The registry is a joint effort involving the FDA, National Heart, Lung, and Blood Institute, Centers for Medicare and Medicaid Services (CMS), and clinicians, scientists, and industry. There is not enough data to show that the indications for continuation is not there.

CORONARY ASSIST DEVICES

Coronary assist devices and mechanical hearts are being developed or perfected to perform the functions of live tissue. Artificial hearts have been under development since the 1950s. In 1966 Dr. DeBakey first successfully implanted a booster pump as a temporary assist device. Columbia's cardiac surgeons have been instrumental in the development of a LVAD (left ventricular assist device)to function as a bridge to transplantation for those waiting for a new heart to become available. Columbia University Medical Center's lead role in the REMATCH clinical trial helped to lead to approval for the LVAD as a permanent, or destination therapy as well. In 1969, Dr. Denton Cooley implanted the first completely artificial heart in a human again on a temporary basis. The first permanent artificial heart, designed by Dr. Robert Jarvik, was implanted in 1982. Numbers of patients have received the Jarvik heart or other artificial hearts since, but surviving recipients have tended to suffer strokes and related problems.

There is a tremendous gap in the number of patients waiting for new hearts and the number of organs that actually become available. In addition to avoiding the immunosuppression and rejection complications of transplantation, success in clinical application of such mechanical devices can help resolve the issue of organ availability. New reparative surgical procedures as alternatives to cardiac transplantation have been described by Lefemine et al (1977) and more recently by a Brazilian inventor Batista which involve cutting away parts of the ventricular wall in enlarged hearts to restore normal proportions and improve performance.

Advances in immunosuppression have most recently involved the development and expanded use of polyclonal and monoclonal antibodies to counteract steroid resistant rejection. Accelerated atherosclerosis in the transplanted heart is believed to be caused or aggravated by the required suppression of the body's normal immunology. Advances in the science of immunology may hold the key to expanding the success of heart transplantation for treatment of end-stage cardiac disease.

CHEST IMPLANTED LVAD

The Heart Ware Ventricular Assist System, a small left ventricular assist device that is implanted in the chest instead of the abdomen has been approved by the Food and Drug Administration as a bridge to heart transplant for the end-stage heart failure patients. The Heartware Ventricular System includes an implantable pump with an external driver and power source. The device is another treatment option for advanced heart failure patients, especially those who are smaller in size or can't have an abdominal implant. The approval of the continuous flow pump device comes less than 3 years after the agency approved Thoratec's HeartMate II left ventricular assist device (LVAD) for destination therapy. That device quickly replaced the previous generation of pulsatile devices. This is the first time that the FDA has approved a ventricular assist device using comparator data from a registry as a control, according to the agency.

The approval was based on data from the ADVANCE trial, which compared the outcomes of 137 patients implanted with the HeartWare System and of patients registered by the Interagency Registry for Mechanically Assisted Circulatory Support (INTERMACS). The registry has been in place since 2005. A total of 140 patients received the investigational pump and 499 patients received a commercially available pump implanted contemporaneously. At 180 days, 90.7% of the investigational pump patients and 90.1% of the of the controls had survived establishing the non-inferiority of the investigational pump. Induction right heart failure, device replacement, stroke, kidney dysfunction, hemolysis, and arrhythmia rates for the HVAD were similar to those reported previously for the HeartMate II.

Results of the ADVANCE trial showed that at 6 months, median 6-minute walk distance were improved by 128.5 meters and functional capacity and quality of life improved markedly and the adverse event profile was favorable. HeartWare registry data facilitated the development and availability of this new device. The registry is a joint effort involving the FDA, National Heart, Lung, and Blood Institute, Centers for Medicare and Medicaid Services (CMS), and clinicians, scientists, and industry. There is not enough data to show that the indications for VADs can be expanded to lower risk patients. Medicare currently does not have an open national coverage determination for VADs. Medicare currently reimburses VADs under certain criteria such as a bridge to transplant and as destination therapy. The 140 U.S. centers that place LVADs are expected to implant nearly 3000 devices this year. Nearly 4,600 patients have received an LVAD since 2010.

Cardiac Interventions assist mechanisms

CHAPTER 9

Cardiac Interventions

ONE WAY TO improve the function of the failed or failing heart besides correcting valvular incompetence or revascularization of the coronary system or adding an LVAD is to change the dynamics of the failed left ventricle. Many of these left ventricles have been damaged as a result of previous myocardial infarction. This is readily identified at catheterization with a left ventriculogram and calculation of the ejection fraction which will fall below 25% and a ventriculogram that will show a feeble contraction. This may happen with or without the presence of an aneurysm. This is the type of heart that VADs are designed for. It is also the type of reduced function that can be helped If you happen to be doing a coronary bypass for coronary occlusion or it may be the primary diagnosis. Sometimes the anterior wall is impaired or even flaccid. There may be the beginning of an aneurysm. This type left ventricle can be improved by a resection of the flaccid or non-contracting anterior wall. These are usually thinned out and the myocardium is replaced by scar or fibrous tissue. Removal of an aneurysmal or thinned out anterior wall will improve the efficiency of the contracting muscle that is left. This will work only if there is functional myocardium remaining posteriorly and laterally. These patients usually will require some form of assisted circulation post operatively and perhaps even in the operating room to get off the bypass. The most commonly available device is the intra-aortic balloon counterpulsator which can safely be used for days after the operation. Left ventricular wall resection for aneurysm and akinesia in 50 consecutive patients was reported by Lefemine et al in the Annals of Thoracic Surgery in 1977. This approach was later presented by Batista (Brazil). The development of Ventricular Assist Device Therapy may overshadow surgical resection as primary therapy. The incidence of heart failure in the United States is about 5.1 million American adults and this figure is projected to increase by 25% by 2030 in individuals over the age of 45. The incidence of heart failure has reached 670,000 new cases each year with more than 56,000 annual deaths due to heart failure. The total cost of treating heart failure in 2012 reached almost $31 billion which is expected to reach $70 billion by 2030. When mechanical circulatory support emerged in the 1980s in an effort to keep patients with post cardiotomy heart failure alive long enough to obtain a donor organ for transplantation the expected survival amounted to days. Survival with these mechanical devices such as HeartMate II Left VentricularAssist System has grown in the last 5 years to a level of 15,000 patients, world wide 6000 of whom are still living. Approximately 300 patients with the HeartMate II device are currently alive with continued support for more than 5 years. Patients are now living longer on these devices. Some patients choose to stay on the VAD and not go the route of transplantation. Time horizons for patients on the VAD is being expanded to horizons of 5 to 10 years. Patients with these devices are just living longer. After the BTT (bridge to transplantation) trial the device is now undergoing trial as destination therapy rather than a bridge to therapy. The role of VADs is now being considered to be included in list of therapies currently available for patients in stage D refractory heart failure. For example some patients are not eligible for transplantation and should be considered for mechanical circulatory support such as a VAD before the patient's heart failure progresses to a terminal, irreversible state. One of the realities to be faced now is that the number of suitable donors for heart transplantation in this country has remained static, and yet the epidemic of heart failure patients is growing at an astronomic pace. Thus there will be a choice to be made for some heart failure patients whether to use VADs as a destination therapy since they may be the only therapy available. The experience to date is in a recent study among patients with a VAD at 1 year after implantation, only 42% of these patients actually received a transplant whereas nearly the same percentage are still alive and doing well waiting for an organ to become available.

The question of Quality of life while being supported by a VAD is important since the wait for a transplant may be extensive. The role of HeartMate II provides some data by reducing adverse events and lowering mortality compared to other generations of VADs. The adverse events problems for patients on VADs include events such as bleeding, infection, cardiac arrhythmias, and hemorrhagic stroke. One of the most feared complications with VAD therapy is stroke which can present as hemorrhagic, ischemic or mixed. Based on published data the stroke rates observed in patients with the HeartMate II device are the lowest reported in a VAD population. Many patients who present with advanced heart disease can barely walk at all; a large proportion are so disabled by heart failure that they are bed- bound. Objective data demonstrate that at 6 months post-implant, patients receiving the HeartMate II device are able to walk an average of 377 yards in a period of 6minutes. Based on recent advances in VAD therapy, we are at a point of having to choose between a VAD and transplantation as options for patients with heart failure. Heart Transplantation is still the gold standard but in Europe, as in the United States a donor heart is becoming a rare asset and patients who want to be considered for transplant have to be in superb condition. In other instances patients patients may need a VAD simply to become a suitable candidate for a transplant in the setting of worsening heart failure or severe pulmonary hypertension. Chronologic age of the patient need not be used as a discriminator for selecting patients for VAD implantation. HeartMate II is a smaller device than HeartMate I and has been implanted in over 100 patients and has been successfully used in patients with a body surface area less than 1.5M2. There seems to be an appropriate time in the course of the disease to implant a VAD, that is before there is multiorgan failure, such as multiple admissions to the hospital for heart failure, and the need to lower doses of heart failure medicines due to lower blood pressure, worsening appetite, and/or weight loss etc. Significant changes in the patients condition for the worse should be the time to talk to the surgeon about implantation of a VAD.

Balloon Angioplasty

Balloon Angioplaasty refers to the technique of inserting a catheter from an arm or femoral artery into a coronary artery and inflated at the point of obstruction whether stenosis by plaque or clot usually caused by plaque and now also includes the placement of a stent from the tip of the catheter which is left in place to keep the artery open after removal of the catheter. A variety of stents are available with or without a heparin coating to prevent clotting early or later. Clotting or obstructing tissue are all too common with this technique and may occur early or late in the course of the disease. This is all performed under local anesthesia, usually through the femoral artery. A guide wire is passed followed by a catheter. The process is all done under fluoroscopy. Placement is verified by dye injection of dye. When the first guide catheter is in place the ballon catheter is placed and inflated briefly as a test. The balloon reaches a diameter of about 1/8 inch. If there is no pain It is inflated for a full minute. About half the patients treated by balloon angioplasty alone will require a repeat procedure at a later date. The patient is treated with prescription drugs to prevent clotting. In the late 1990s about 500,000 people underwent angioplasty.

There is a long history for this procedure as usual. Werner Forsmann was the first known doctor to enter the heart with a catheter. This of course led to diagnostic heart catheterization that is now routine before heart surgery. An Oregon doctor, Charles Dotter investigated dilatation of narrowed arteries by means of catheters in the 1960s. The balloon concept was developed in 1973 at the University Hospital of Zurich in Switzerland. They, Porstmann and Gruentzig are credited with performing the first balloon angioplasty to open a clogged artery. Gruentzig later emigrated to the US and died ina plane crash in 1985. Within 10 years of the introduction of this technique of coronary dilatation it was being performed over 200,000 times a year and it has grown and been refined with the introduction of stainless steel stents, newer balloons, newer materials, and better anticoagulation during and after the procedure. There is no need to discus the advantages of whether to use the radial artery versus the femoral artery. There is evidence that there is less blood loss using the radial artery in women. Compared with men women have an increased risk of bleeding from anti-thrombotic therapy as well as femoral access. About 40% of patients who have balloon angioplasty are at risk of more blockages in the treated area and usually it happens within 6 months after balloon angioplasty. Even with stents about 20% will have restenosis. Newer designs are always in the works. smaller stents, coated stents and and recently non-metal stents that will dissolve into the artery.

CORONARY ANGIOPLASTY

A large portion of heart disease, death and disability is the result not of valve disease or dysfunction but of coronary disease which results from narrowing or total occlusion of one or more coronary arteries. This can result in a number of complications, death, negative changes of the anatomy of the heart and symptoms that are debilitating and painful. There is little question that heart disease not only can cause a variety of symptoms but they can be reduced in incidence, controlled by medicines, reduced by proper diet, medical and surgical treatment, and even replaced on a temporary or permanent basis. The pharmacology associated with treatment is extensive and effective. Prevention of disease has been a hallmark of medicine for many years especially if you know the cause of the problem e.g. penicillin in rheumatic disease, cholesterol in diets. This is not a medical treatise and some items may not be mentioned. Everyone is aware of the ekg and radiology but may not know the extent of radiology in diagnosing abnormalities in the coronaries, but also abnormalities of the wall as well as the state of function of the remaining wall. It will pinpoint the point of obstruction or occlusion as the case maybe but current arteriography makes it possible to treat many of these lesions with stents of varying design such as a mesh with heparin attached or some other anticoagulant, or relieves obstruction in a supporting channel that relieves not only the ischemia but salvages the possibility of damage to the myocardium. A large portion of heart disease, death and disability is not valve disease or dysfunction but coronary disease which results from narrowing or total occlusion of one or more coronary arteries. This can result in a number of complications, death, negative changes of the anatomy of the heart and symptoms that are debilitating and painful. There are complications such as limited life span, and sources of thrombosis that account for the need for anticoagulation. Many variations of operations have been devised in attempts by the surgical profession to treat or at least relieve the limitations imposed by coronary obstruction. It was one of the most accessible of diseases because it was on the surface of the heart. The atheromata were often visible but the surgeons did not have the techniques. A number of treatments were tried for relieving the pain and the disability. Thes included thyroidectomy, pericardial adhesions, radioactive iodine, attaching a pectoral muscle to the heart. O'Shaughnessy published a report in 1938 relatingthe degenerative changes in the myocardium to the sclerosis in the arteries. But in his operation he only sutured the omentum to the pericardium though he had put aleuronat paste between the heart and the pericardium and reported 20 cases. Five died one was free of angina, he never publish another article. Fauteux in 1940 reported on the effect of ligating the Magna Cordis vein. The interested surgeons decided that the beneficial effects were not great enough to continue. In 1941 Robertson et al published a paper on experimental coronary sinus obstruction. Heinbecker tried placing an irritant in the pericardium. These were all a part of a grand effort to improve the blood supply to the heart on both cotinents. A different method for creating a new blood supply was described by Vineberg in 1946. He transplanted the left internal mammary artery into the wall of the left ventricle. He was able to demonstrate an anastomosis between the internal mammary artery and the left coronary artery. In 1948 he published the results of further experiments which he did in 3 parts. And demonstrated a connection between the left internal mammary artery with multiple connections and vascularization of the surrounding tissue. His last article indicated that he had done the operation on 1500 dogs. Litwak finally did experiments with constriction of the coronary arteries. Though five of the dogs died within 5 weeks but injection of Schlesinger solution showed internal mammary connection in three of them. Six dogs that lived more than 5 months demonstrated an anastomosis between the coronary arteries and the internal mammary artery and the entire left ventricle. Vineberg had operated on 59 patients since 1950. Seventeen had angina at rest and there was an operative mortality of 59%.

It became obvious that the procedures that were being tested were inadequate for the need. Rene Favaloro after receiving his medical degree in Argentina in 1949 became interested in cardiovascular interventions and developed an enthusiasm for thoracic surgery and he ended up at the Cleveland Clinic as a resident and later as a member of the surgery team working with Donald Effler then head of cardiovascular surgery. Also with Mason Sones who was in charge of angiography laboratory and William Proudfit who was head of cardiology. In the beginning his work revolved around valvular and congenital diseases. He would spend hours reviewing coronary angiograms and studying coronary arteries and their relation to cardiac muscle. Sones was the father of coronary angiography and had a huge collection of angiograms. At the beginning of 1967 Favaloro began to consider the possibility of using the saphenous vein in coronary surgery. He did his first case in May of 1967 and in 1970 published the first volume of "Surgical Treatment of Coronary Arteriosclerosis "This became a world wide phenomenon with thousands of cases being done at all major and even minor cardiac surgical centers. His contributions to teaching by talks and participation in seminars was phenomenal and he went to Argentina to establish the Favaloro Foundation which he did with his own money. In 1980 came the Laboratorio de Investigation Basica which he financed and this later became "The University Institute of Biomedical Sciences." In 1990, later transformed to Universidd Favaloro (1998). In 1992 came the non-profit Favaloro Foundation Institute of Cardiology and Cardiovascular Surgery with many highly specialized services.

BYPASS SURGERY STATISTICS

Bypass surgery is a major operation done because there are symptoms of chest pain or a heart attack or increasing disability with angina and shortness of breath with exercise indicating blockage of the arterial supply to the heart. Workup will usually include cardiac catheterization most importantly coronary angiograms to pinpoint the degree of coronary blockage and the specific arteries that need bypass. The operation under consideration is coronary artery bypass a very major operation that carries a risk to life and a risk of complications. Now there is an alternate option which will be described in detail in another section, done in the catheterization laboratory by trained cardiologists. Thousands of coronary bypasses have been done since its introduction in 1967 and there is a body of knowledge and experience even though the coronary angioplasty has reduced the number of coronary bypasses being done.

Risk of death during during the bypass or during the hospitalization is 2-4%

Stroke occurs in 1-2%

In 5-10% of coronary artery bypass grafts, the graft fails and stops flowing blood. The annual mortality for patients with 2 or 3 vessel disease who are treated conservatively with appropriate medication is less than 1% a year.

In 17,857 patients with disease of all three arteries who underwent coronary artery bypass surgery, the annual mortality rate was 3.3%. In 1,294 patients with three vessel disease who underwent coronary angioplasty the annual mortality rate was 4.2%.

In 9,212 patients with two vessel disease undergoing coronary artery bypass surgery, the annual mortality rate was 2.7%. In 7,405 patients with two vessel disease undergoing coronary angioplasty the annual mortality rate was 2.3%.

Dr Salem Yusuf reviewed the medical literature from 1972 to 1984 and compared the mortality of medical and surgical treatment There were four studies involving 416 patients. At 10 years the mortality of the surgically treated patients was 33% or 3.3% per year. The mortality of the medically treated patients at 10 years was 34% or 3.4% per year. This represents the medical treatment primarily of the Seventies.

Dr Spencer King of Emory University compared 194 bypass surgery patients with 198 angioplasty patients. The annual mortality for bypass surgery patients was 2.1% and that for the angioplasty patients was 2.4% per year.

Ages	Mortality after Angioplasty		Mortality after Bypass Surgery	
	30 day	1year	30 day	1 year
	%	%	%	%
65-69	2.1	5.2	4.3	8.0
70-74	3.0	7.3	5.7	10.6
75-79	4.6	10.9	7.4	14.2
80+	7.8	17.3	10.9	19.5

Mortality rate is related to age

From the University of Washington comes a study of the 15 year survival rate of the coronary artery surgery Study of 6,018 men and 1,095 women who originally underwent treatment between 1974 and 1979. For medical treatment the 15 year survival rate for men was 50% and 49% for women. For those with initial surgical treatment the survival for men was 52% and 48% for women. Thus there was no significant difference in survival between the two treatments with the annual mortality being 3.3%.

Another study was the Caveat trial (Coronary Angioplasty Versus Excisional Atherectomy Trial) Atherectomy refers to the use of a rotor rooter type of device that is inserted into a coronary artery and the atherosclerotic plaque is cut up and scooped out. In this study only the frequency of a myocardial infarction (heart attack) was studied in 500 patients undergoing angioplasty and 512 having atherectomy. The incidence of myocardial infarction in the atherectomy patients was 15.2% and it was 6.8% in the angioplasty patients. The high incidence of heart attacks with both groups was because cardiac enzymes were measured rather than merely getting an electrocardiogram after the procedure.

Another study dealing with mortality rate in elderly patients undergoing cardiac surgery is from Cedars-Sinai Medical Center in Los Angeles. In a study of 528 patients over 80, the 30 day mortality was 8.3%. At one year it was 18% and at 5 years 38%. From the St. Louis University Health Sciences center a review of 250 Patients undergoing coronary artery bypass surgery found that the annual mortality for patients between 60 and 79 was about 7% per year and for patients above the age of 80 it was 13% per year.

From the Mass General Hospital in a trial 127 patients undergoing angioplasty or coronary bypass surgery the annual cardiovascular event rate was 7.7 per year for the surgery patients and 17.7% per year for angioplasty patients.

From the Thoraxcenter at Erasmus university in Rotterdam a 10 year study of 856 patients undergoing angioplasty revealed an annual mortality rate of 2.2% and an annual cardiovascular event rate of 8.6%.

In the BARI trial (Bypass Angioplasty Revascularization Investigation) 1829 patients were followed for 5.4 years. Annual mortality was 2.1% per year for bypass surgery and 2.7% per year for angioplasty. Event rate was 4% per year for surgery and 4.3% per year for angioplasty.

In a 10 year study from St. Antonius Hospital in the Netherlands, 351 patients who had angioplasty were followed. Annual mortality was 2% and cardiovascular event rate 10% per year.

From the University of North Carolina at Greensboro, 633 patients who were treated with primary angioplasty for their heart attack were followed for 5.3 years. The in-hospital mortality was very high at 9% and the cardiac mortality at 5 years was another 9%. Total mortality was twice what it should have been.

From the University of Ottawa Heart Institute in Ontario Canada a 25 year study of 1,388 patients who underwent bypass surgery at an average age of only 48 years reveals an annual mortality of 2%. Eighteen Percent had to-undergo repeat surgery during this period.

From the Veterans Affairs Medical Center and the University of Colorado Health Sciences Center in Denver comes a study of 131 patients above the age of 70 with unstable angina who underwent coronary angioplasty for their symptoms, the mortality at 30 days was a striking 13%

In a comparison of medical treatment versus angioplasty for patients with stable coronary disease, 20 centers from the united kingdom and Ireland treated 1018 patients. The risk of death or a heart attack was 2.3% per year for angioplasty treated patients but only 1.2% per year for medically treated patients.

In a recent Veterans Administration study known as VANQWISH trial 920 patients from 15 medical centers with an acute heart attack were randomized to treatment with revascularization (angioplasty or coronary artery bypass surgery) or conservative medical treatment. At the time of discharge from the hospital, 21 patients who had undergone revascularization had died versus only six medically treated patients. At 2.5 years there were 80 deaths in the treated group versus only 59 deaths in the conservatively treated patients.

There are only a few reports dealing with the use of stents placed within a coronary artery. A stent is a metal tube that can be expanded when placed in a coronary artery. When fully expanded it becomes a scaffolding that helps to keep the artery from closing. Typically, when an artery is dilated with balloon angioplasty, a delayed complication is ccollapse of the walls of the blood vessel causing the artery to become blocked. Stents were developed to keep this from happening This it does and although it does this successfully the inside of the stent becomes filled with tissue that grows into the stent. Thus stents often become occluded and the vessel still closes off.

From Harvard University comes a report on 175 patients who had stents inserted. Annual mortality was 2.7% and the annual cardiovascular event rate was 14.7%per year

IS THE PATIENT BETTER?

It is apparent from the many reports that the mortality rate as well as other complications of coronary bypass surgery and angioplasty vary considerably and outcome depends in large measure upon the patients age, how much heart disease is present, the skill of the doctor who is treating the patient and many other factors. What is clear is that there is no advantage of either surgery or angioplasty over medical treatment. There is no evidence that either of these two procedures will prevent heart attacks or premature death. Furthermore do these procedures cause any harm? The answer to this question is not clear. A sizable number of imaging studies using echocardiogram, radioactive imaging, and (PET) positron emission tomography, have not clarified the basic question. To complicate matters, imaging done immediately after revascularization will usually show impaired function. If however the imaging study is delayed for several months, recovery will often be seen. It is clear that recovery will occur without any treatment. This occurs through the hearts own revascularization process with the development of new vessels into the area where the coronaries are narrowed or blocked.

A recent report from the department of cardiology at the Academic Hospital in Leiden in the Netherlands has reviewed 37 studies using a variety of imaging procedures. Improvement after revascularization occurred only 37-55% of the time the remainder of the hearts were either no better or worse. There seems to be no way of predicting the result in the individual patient. Those who showed no viable muscle after a heart attack were less likely to show improvement, And those with viable muscle often did not show improvement.

Both coronary by-pass surgery and angioplasty will relieve recurring chest pain in subjects with coronary artery disease. In the case of bypass surgery 10-20% do not get effective relief while patients who receive angioplasty will have a return of their symptoms in 40-50%. However, relief of pain will occur in 75% of patients without any treatment within 3-6 months. Medication will speed things up and relieve pain in an additional 20% with a far lower complication rate

CHAPTER 10

Heart Transplantation

PIONEERING MEDICAL AND surgical research conducted from the late 1700s until the early 1900s set the stage in the field of immunology that evolved into today's transplantation successes. Among the notable breakthroughs were Ehrlich's discovery of antibodies and antigens, Landsteiner's blood typing, and Metchnikoffs theory of host resistance. Advances in suturing techniques in the 19th century allowed surgeons to transplant organs in the laboratory. By the 20th century transplants invariably failed because transplants between species and even between the same species (xenographic and allogenic transplants) invariably failed while autografts (within the same individual, like skin grafts) were almost always successful. It was understood that repeat transplants between the same donor and recipient experienced accelerated rejection and success was more likely when the donor and recipient shared a "blood relationship."

Alexis Carrel was a French surgeon and Nobel Laureate whose experiments involved sustaining life in animal organs outside the body. He received the Nobel Prize in 1912 for his technique for suturing blood vessels in animal organs outside the body. In the 1930s he collaborated with the aviator Charles Lindbergh to invent a mechanical heart that circulated vital fluids through excised organs. Various organs and animal tissues were kept alive for many years in this way. Throughout the 1940s and 50s small advances were made and Andre Cournaud and Dickinson Richards were awarded the same Nobel prize in physiology for their contributions to an understanding of the human heart using cardiac catheterization. Keith Reemtsma showed that imunnosuppressive drugs would prolong heart transplant survival in the laboratory setting. At this time, Norman Shumway, Richard Lower and their associates at Stanford were embarking on the development of heart-lung machines and solving perfusion problems and correction of heart valve defects and experimenting with topical hypothermia which could give the surgeons a blood -free environment and time to perform repairs. Next came autotransplantation where the heart was excised and resutured back in place. By the mid 1960s immunological rejection was the only remaining impediment to clinical heart transplantation.

In 1967, a human heart from one person was transplanted into the body of another by a South African surgeon named Dr. Christian Barnard in Cape Town. He removed the heart of a 25 year old woman who died following an auto accident and placed it in the chest of Louis Washkanski, a 55 year old man dying of heart damage. The patient survived for 18 days. Dr Barnard had studied with the Shumway group and learned most of his technique from them. This generated world wide interest and acclaim. The patient died of a pulmonary infection less than 3 weeks postoperatively. More than 100 transplants were performed in 1968 but the results were dismal. By 1970 fewer than 20 transplants were done. And the majority of these were done at the Stanford University Medical Center. There has been an improvement both in the number and quality since those early days and more than 350 human cardiac transplants performed at Stanford since those early days. And the factors that made it possible were the selection of patients and as well as the development of a number of very effective immunosuppressive agents such as cyclosporine. Techniques for procuring donors from distant sites enlarge the pool greatly and has made cardiac transplantation a daily reality. Appropriate candidates fall into two pools: those with end-stage coronary disease and those with cardiomyopathy usually less than 55 years of age. There are strict criteria used for the selection of a suitable donor such as the donor should be less than 35 years of age and not have been subject to prolonged resuscitative procedures. The recipient should not be more than 20% larger and be of the same ABO blood group. Infection and rejection remain the biggest causes of morbidity and mortality. Graft atherosclerosis remains a common problem. Approximately half the patients will experience an episode of rejection during the first postoperative month and 80% wii experience it after the first 3 months. Another major problem is graft atherosclerosis.

Sometimes re-transplantation has been necessary. Lympho-reticular disease and arrhythmias are occasionally seen in the longterm survivors.

Cardiac transplantation continues to be the ultimate treatment for many patients with end-stage heart failure in spite of the increasing availability of rotary blood pumps for implantation. After orthotopic heart transplantation combination immunosuppressive therapy is necessary to control the potential complications of acute cellular rejection and antibody mediated (humeral)rejection which frequently necessitates plasmapheresis. Chronic cardiac rejection is characterized by coronary allograft vasculopathy, which is mediated by immunologic mechanisms that involve alloimmune and autoimmune processes in addition to many nonimmunity related donor and recipient factors. Coronary allograft vasculopathy is the leading indication for repeat transplantation in some patients. Cardiogenic shock accompanying the acute rejection of a transplanted heart is an unusual but life threatening occurance. In this situation mechanical circulatory support has been recognized as an important method of short-term support while the immunotherapy is adjusted to control the acute rejection. There are reports of recovery after the application of mechanical circulatory support for severe post- transplant rejection with cardiogenic shock 7 months after transplantation. The process of treatment (Caceres and colleagues) consisted of intraortic balloon, then extracorporeal membrane oxygenation followed by implantation of a bi-ventricular assist device (Thoratec corp.) No further episodes of severe acute rejection were observed at one year followup.

In 1984 the world's first successful pediatric heart transplant was performed at Columbia Medical Center on a 4 year old boy. He received a second transplant in 1989 and continues to live a productive life. In 1984 in Loma Linde, California, Leonard Bailey, MD implanted a baboon heart into a 12-day-old girl. The infant survived for 20 days. In 1994 a new drug, tacrolimus or FK-506, also derived from a fungus, was approved for immunosuppression.

CARDIOPULMONARY HOMOTRANSPLANTATION

There is a long-standing interest in cardiopulmonary transplantation though the clinical results have been disappointing. Cyclosporin and the clinical results in non- primates has spurred the interest in applying this technique to a population of patients with end-stage pulmonary vascular disease and pulmonary parenchymal disease resistant to medical therapy or management. The changes associated with pulmonary vascular pathology may not be apparent and become irreversible. Early experience included patients with primary pulmonary hypertension and ccongenital heart disease. The early experience was generally disappointing because of difficulties with bronchial anastomosis, rejection, infection, denervation, interruption of lymphatics and respiratory failure. Because of the broad spectrum of potential candidates for cardiopulmonary transplantation it has been necessary to limit the initial program to young patients with end-stage cardiopulmonary disease. Other potential indications include chronic airway obstruction with cor pulmonale, interstitial pulmonary disease including pulmonary fibrosis and sarcoidosis. A principal limitation to a broader application of heart-lung transplantation is the availability of suitable donors. The criteria for donors includes maintaining a po2 greater than lOOon 30% oxygen, No radiographic evidence of pulmonary disease, and a peak inspiratory pressure of less than 30 mm hg. Maintenance of the heart-lung donor is more critical because the need for preservation of pulmonary function so it is necessary to manipulate fluid administration and peripheral resistance and to procure the graft as soon as possible after declaration of brain death. The donor portion is done without cardiopulmonary bypass. A standard potassium cardioplegic solution is used to treat the heart and a modified Collins solution is used to preserve the lungs and the whole specimen is preserved by cooling. In the recipient great effort is used to preserve the the vagi nerves, the phrenic nerves, and the recurrent laryngeal nerve. Topical and injected cold solution is used in the specimen during the implantation. Tracheal anastomosis comes next and is preferred over bronchial anastomosis. Topical hypothermia as well as infusion hypothermia is used throughout the procedure. Postoperative immunosuppression is similar to that used for cardiac transplant with cyclosporine and azathioprine, and antithymocyte globulin. Steroids are omitted the first two weeks. Baldwin and Shumway reported that 15 of 25 patients survived for 2 to 50 months.

LUNG TRANSPLANTATION

The first human lung transplant was performed by Hardy on June 11,1963 in a patient with chronic lung disease and carcinoma of the left lung. The patient survived 18 days before dying of renal insufficiency. Patient and donor must reside in the same institution in order to minimize donor lung ischemia, bronchial anastomosis complications, and allograft rejection. Only 38 lung transplants were performed in the first 15 years of clinical experience. The longest survivor was a 23 year old sandblaster with micro nodular silicosis who lived 10 months after allograft transplantation. The American College of Surgeons Organ Transplant Registry (1975) recorded 36 clinical lung transplants with no patient living longer than 10 months. Some current statistics as of 2008 are as follows

	1 YEAR SURVIVAL	5 YEARS SURVIVAL	10 YEARS SURVIVAL
LUNG TRANSPLANT	83.6%	53.4%	28.4%
HEART-LUNG TRANSPLANT	73.8%	46.5%	28.3%

Transplanted lungs typically last 3 to 5 years before showing signs of failure.

While lung transplants carry risk as indicated on the table above, they also extend life expectancy and particulary enhance the quality of life for end-stage pulmonary patients. It was after the invention of the heart-lung machine coupled with the development of immunosuppressive drugs such as cyclosporine that organs like the lungs could be transplanted with a reasonable chance of recovery.

The first successful transplant surgery involving the lungs was a heart-lung transplant performed by Dr. Bruce Reitz of Stanford University on a woman who had idiopathic pulmonary hypertension.

- 1983: First successful long-term single lung transplant (Tom Hall) by Joel Cooper (Toronto)
- 1986 First successful long-term double-lung transplant (Ann Harrison) by Joel Cooper (Toronto)
- 1988: First successful long-term double-lung transplant for cystic fibrosis by Joel Cooper (Toronto)

There are special requirements for both candidate for lung transplant and for the recipient. It is important that the donor be of the same blood type as the recipient because rejection is more likely and more severe. Obviously health status of the donor should be good and lung size should be a fit. For the recipient there is a long list that includes end-stage lung disease that does not respond to any therapy and does not have other chronic or infectious disease. Bad habits such as drug use, smoking, or inability to comply with a rigorous post-transplant regimen of medications as well as continuing medical care would be against having the operation which carries major risk and is a very large undertaking. The candidate for a lung will be subject a large number of medical tests such as tissue typing, x-rays, CT scanning, pulmonary function tests, stress tests, ventilation tests, cardiac catheterization, echocardiogram, bone density, and probably others. Even after passing all these tests there is a lung allocation score that the recipient is subject to. It is no longer a first come first serve system, but each recipient older than 12 years is given a lung allocation score or LAS which takes into account various measures of the patients health. Patients under 12 are given priority.

Patients who are accepted as good potential transplant candidates must carry a pager with them in case a good donor organ becomes available. These patients must be prepared to move to their transplant center at a moments notice and to limit their travel.

TYPES OF LUNG TRANSPLANT

Many patients can be helped by the transplantation of a single healthy lung, usually obtained from a donor that has been pronounced brain dead. The double lung transplant is usually performed in patients with cystic fibrosis because of the bacterial colonization of the recipients lungs. Some recipients also have severe cardiac disease and for them there is the possibility perhaps the necessity of a heart-lung transplant. We should mention the so-called 'domino' transplant first performed in 1987 in which a heart-lung transplant is performed in a patient whose healthy heart is then transplanted into another patient waiting for a heart transplant. It takes about an hour to prepare the patient, the surgeon inspects the donor lung for defects general anesthesia is induced and the appropriate incision for single or double lung is made. A double lung transplant, also known as a bilateral transplant, can be executed sequentially, en bloc, or simultaneously. Sequential is more common effectively like having two single – lung transplants done. Bronchoscopy is performed after the first transplant. The patient will be cared for in the intensive care unit for a few days, average hospital stay is one to three weeks, with complications longer, and then discharged to a rehabilitation gym for approximately three months to regain fitness. Other side effects are that the patient cannot feel the need or the urge to cough, or feel when their lungs are congested. They must therefore make conscious effort to deepbreath and cough. Other possible changes are that the heart rate responds less quickly because the vagus nerve is cut there may be a change in their voice due to damage to nerves that control voice. All recipients are kept from driving for three months.

Hygiene becomes very important because of the Immunosuppressant drugs which are required every day. The number of possible complications after this kind of surgery is long. Transplant rejection becomes a primary concern and continues for the rest of life. Usually the immunosuppressive regimen starts right after surgery, and usually indudes cyclosporine, azathioprine and sometimes tacrolimus is given instead of cyclosporine and mofetil instead of azathioprine. Infection becomes a prime concern and must be treated with antibiotics. Chronic rejection meaning repeated bouts of rejection occurs in about 50% of patients.

CHAPTER 11

LUNG TRANSPLANTATION

- Lung transplantation or pulmonary transplantation is a surgical procedure in which a patients diseased lungs are partially or totally replaced by lungs which come from a donor. While lung transplants carry certain associated risks they can also extend life expectancy and enhance the the quality of life for end-stage pulmonary patients. Lung transplantation is the therapeutic measure of last resort for patients who have end- stage lung disease and have exhausted all other available treatments without improvement. A variety of conditions may make such surgery necessary. The most common reasons for lung transplantation in the United States were:
- Chronic obstructive disease (copd)
- Pulmonary fibrosis
- Cystic fibrosis
- Idiopathic pulmonary hypertension
- Alpha 1-antitrypsin deficiency
- Replacing previously transplanted lungs

Other causes are bronchiectasis and sarcoidosis. Contraindications are:

- Concurrent chronic illness e.g. heart failure, kidney disease, liver disease
- Current infections including HIV and Hepatitis
- Current or recent cancer
- Current use of alcohol, tobacco, or illegal drugs

- Age
- Psychiatric conditions
- History of non-compliance with instructions

The history of organ transplants began with several attempts that were unsuccessful due to transplant rejection. Animal experiments by various pioneers, including Vladimir Demikhov and Dominique Metras during the 1940s and the 1950s first demonstrated that the procedure was technically feasible. James Hardy of the University of Mississippi perfomed the first human lung transplant on June 11,1963. Following a single-lung transplantation the patient, identified later as convicted murderer John Richard Russell survived for eighteen days. From 1963 to 1978, multiple attempts at lung transplantation failed because of rejection and problems with anastomotic bronchial healing. It was only after the invention of the heart-lung machine, coupled with the development of immunosuppressive drugs such as cyclosporine that organs such as the lungs could be transplanted with a reasonable chance of patient recovery.

- The first successful transplant surgery involving the lungs was a heart-lung transplant performed by Dr. Bruce Reitz of Stanford University on a woman who had idiopathic pulmonary hypertension.
- 1983 The first successful long-term single lung transplant (Tom Hall) by Joel Cooper (Toronto)
- 1986 The first successful long-term double lung transplant (Ann Harrison)by Joel Cooper (Toronto)
- 1988 The first successful long-term double -lung transplantfor cystic fibrosis by Joel Cooper (Toronto)

Transplant Requirements
Requirements for potential donors
There are certain requirements for the donor of a lung or two lungs

- Healthy
- Size match
- Age
- Blood type

There are requirements for potential recipients. These are generally agreed upon

- End-stage lung disease
- Exhausted other available therapies
- No other chronic medical condition
- No current infections or recent cancer
- No HIV or hepatitis
- No alcohol, smoking, or drug abuse
- An acceptable weight range
- Age
- Acceptable psychological profile
- Has social support system
- Financially able to pay for expenses
- Able to comply with post-transplant regimen

Patients who are to undergo lung transplant will have a work-up that seems exhaustive. They will have blood typing, tissue typing, in addition to CT scans, cardiac stress tests, bone scans, standard x-rays of lungs for size, cardiac catheterization, echocardiograms, Ventilation tests, MUGA scans and electrocardiograms. This is probably not the total list.

Having obtained and passed all the tests merely puts you in line with all those who are waiting for a lung or two lungs. The lung allocation system now evaluates the prospective recipients by assigning a lung allocation score or LAS which takes into account various measures of the patients health and need rather than how long they have been on the list. The length of time on the list may be used as a deciding factor when when there are others with the same score. These eligible candidates must carry a pager with them at all times in case a donor organ becomes available. Such patients are encouraged to limit their travel within a certain geographical area.

CHAPTER 12

TYPES OF LUNG TRANSPLANT

A LOBE TRANSPLANT IS a surgery in which part of a living donors lung is removed and used to replace part of a recipients diseased lung. This procedure usually involves the donation of lobes from two different people, thus replacing a single lung in the recipient.

A single lung transplant typically comes from a donor who has been pronounced brain-dead

A double lung transplant usually occurs in people with cystic fibrosis due to the bacterial contamination commonly found within such patients lungs. If only one lung is transplanted, bacteria in the native lung could potentially infect the new lung.

A heart-lung transplant is used if there is severe cardiac disease which would necessitate a heart transplant as well as a lung transplant. There is a maneuver called the "domino transplant" which typically involves the transplant of a heart and lungs into recipient A, and whose own healthy heart is removed and transplanted into recipient B.

We will not review the technical details of the operation for either lung or heart and leave that to the surgical team. Obviously it is a long and complex series of maneuvers for the surgeon and his team. The heart-lung transplant requires the heart-lung machine to keep the patient alive while the transfer of organs is accomplished and all organs are sutured in place.

The postoperative care follows the usual routine. The patient may require assisted ventilation for a period of time, iv nutrition will be continued till the patient can tolerate drink.

ASSISTED CIRCULATION

With all these activities repairing and replacing hearts it is natural that these same groups would be interested in mechanisms to assist the heart on a temporary or permanent basis. One of the first to see the need and develop a mechanical apparatus to do this was the arterial counterpulsator developed in Dwight Harken's dog laboratory by Roy H Clauss et al with the help of engineer w. Cliff Birtwell and reported in 1961. It was called the arterial counterpulsator because the mechanism of assisting the heart was to have a catheter in the aorta that would counter pulsate blood that is it would aspirate part of the ejection fraction (systole) and return the aspirated blood during the diastolic period. In other words the work of the heart would be reduced during systole by reducing peripheral resistance and returned during diastole without affecting cardiac output. The aim was to reduce the work of the failing heart on a continuous basis for an indefinite period of time and support the failing heart before surgery if that was the need or after surgery if the heart required temporary support. This could be continued for an indefinite period as required. A machine was constructed and the original is still in a museum. Unfortunately it did not receive extensive use because of a hemolysis problem. However the principal upon which it was based was transferred to use of an intra-aortic balloon that could be introduced via a femoral artery. This was introduced by A Kantrowitz et al and reported in 1968. It has since been accepted as one of the few mechanisms still available to the cardiac surgeon and patient that needs assistance before and after surgery and can be applied quickly on short notice. The balloon is activated by helium and synchronized to deflate during systole and inflate during diastole. It is often referred to as the IABC. Cleveland, Lefemine et al reported its use in 60 patients in 1975 for pre and post operative assistance for days.

CARDIAC ASSSIST DEVICES

A ventricular assist device(VAD) is a mechanical circulatory device that is used to partially or completely replace the function of the failing heart. Some VADs are intended for short term use (months or years) in patients, typically for patients recovering from heart attacks or heart surgery, while others are intended for long-term use (months to years and in some cases for life) typically for patients suffering from advanced congestive failure. VADs are distinct from artificial hearts which are designed to completely take over cardiac function and generally require the removal of the patients heart. VADs are designed to assist either the right (RVAD) or the left(LVAD) ventricle, or both at once (BiVAD). The type that is used depends primarily on the underlying heart disease and the pulmonary arterial resistance that determines the load on the right ventricle. LVADs are most commonly used, but when pulmonary arterial resistance is high right ventricular assistance may become necessary. Long term VADs are normally used to keep patients alive with a good quality of life while they wait for a heart transplantation (known as a bridge to transplantation. However, LVADs are sometimes used as destination therapy, meaning, that they will never undergo heart transplantation, and sometimes as a bridge to recovery. In the last few years, VADs have improved significantly in terms of providing survival and quality of life among recipients.

The pumps used in VADs are divided into two main categories- pulsatile pumps that mimic the natural pulsing action of the heart and continuous flow pumps. Pusatile VADs are positive displacement pumps. In some of these pumps, the volume occupied by blood varies during the pumping cycle, and if the pump is contained inside the body then a vent tube to the outside air is required. Continuous flow VADs are smaller and have proven to be more durable than pulsatile VADs. They normally use either a centrifugal pump or an axial flow pump. Both types have a central rotor containing permanent magnets. Controlled electric currents running through coils contained in the pump housing apply forces to the magnets which in turn cause the rotors to spin. In the centrifugal pumps, the rotors are shaped to accelerate the blood circumferentially and thereby cause it to move toward the outer rim of the pump, whereas in the axial flow pumps the rotors are more or less cylindrical with blades that are helical, causing the blood to be accelerated in the direction of the rotors axis. An important issue with continuous flow pumps is the method used to suspend the rotor. Early versions used solid bearings, however newer pumps some of which are approved for use in the EU, either use Electromagnetic suspension or hydrodynamic suspension. These pumps contain only one moving part.

HISTORY The early VADs emulated the heart by using a pulsatile action in which blood is alternately sucked into the pump from the left ventricle then forced out into the aorta. Devices of this kind include the HeartMate IP LVAS, which was approved for use in the US by the Food and Drug Administration in October 1994. These devices are commonly referred to as first generation VADs. More recent work has concentrated on continuous flow pumps, which can be roughly categorized as either centrifugal pumps or axial flow impellar driven pumps. These pumps have the advantage of greater simplicity resulting in smaller size and greater reliability. These are referred to as second generation VADs. A side effect is that the user will not have a pulse. Or that the pulse intensity will be seriously reduced. Third generation VADs suspend the impeller in the pump using either hydrodynamic or electromagnetic suspension thus removing the need for bearings and reducing the number of moving parts to one. Another technology undergoing clinical trials is the use of trans cutaneous induction to power and control the device rather than using percutaneous cables. This reduces the risk of infection and the consequent need to take preventive action. A pulsatile pump using this technology has CE Mark approval and is in clinical trials for US FDA approval. A very different approach in the early stages of development is the use of an inflatable cuff around the aorta. Inflating the cuff contracts the aorta and deflating the allows the aorta to expand-in effect the aorta becomes a second left ventricle. This approach Harkens back to what may have been the original cardiac assist device that was developed by the Harken group at the Peter Bent Brigham Hospital and reported by Clauss et al in The Journal of Thoracic and Cardiovascular Surgery 1961. The Counterpulsator. The original counterpulsator designed and constructed by Cliff Birtwell an engineer for the Davol company utilized the principal of a cannula in the femoral artery or aorta and an external ventricle that could be synchronized with the contractions of the heart. This ventricle would aspirate blood from the aorta when systolic contraction occurred to reduce the work load of the heart and pump the blood back to the aorta in diastole. This principle was later applied in another design introduced by Kantrowitz which was an arterial counterpulsator using a balloon introduced to the upper aorta which would inflate and deflate a balloon synchronized to the ekg such that it deflated during systole and inflated during diastole to reduce the work of the heart. This kind of apparatus is still available and in use today to assist the failing heart after surgery and sometimes to assist the patient before surgery if there are signs of left ventricular failure.

Peter Houghton was the longest surviving recipient of a VAD for permanent use. He received an experimental Jarvick 2000 LVAD. Since then, he completed a 91 mile charity walk published two books, lectured widely, hiked in the Swiss Alps, and the American West flew an ultralight aircraft and traveled around the world. He died of acute renal failure at the age of 69.

- Some recent experience in assisted circulation: In July 2009 in England surgeons removed a donor heart that had been implanted in a toddler next to her native heart after her native heart had recovered. This shows that it is possible to provide mechanical or biological assistance on a temporary basis to allow a native heart to heal.
- In July 2009,18- month follow-up results from the HeartMate II Clinical Trial concluded that continuous flow LVAD provides effective hemodynamic support for at least 18 months in patients awaiting transplantation, with improved functional status and quality of life.
- Heidelberg University Hospital reported in July 2009 that the first HeartAssistS was implanted there. The HeartAassistS weighs 92 grams is made of titanium and plastic and serves to pump blood from the left ventricle to the aorta.
- A phase one clinical trial is underway (as of August 2009) consisting of patients with coronary bypass and patients in end-stage heart failure who have a left ventricular assist device. The trial involves testing a patch, called Anginera ™ that contains cells that secrete hormone- like growth factors that stimulate other cells to grow. The patches are seeded with heart muscle

cells and the implanted onto the heart with the goal of getting the muscle cells to start communicating with native tissues in a way that allows for regular contractions
- In September 2009, a New Zealand news outlet, Stuff, reported that in another 18 months to two years, a new wireless device will be ready for clinical trial that will power VADs without direct contact. If successful this may reduce the chance of infection as a result of now needing a power cable through the skin for powering the VADs.
- The National Institutes of Health (NIH) awarded a $2.8 million grant to develop a "pulse-less total artificial heart using two VADs by Micromed, initially created by Michael DeBakey and George Noon. The grant was renewed for a second year of research in August 2009. The total artificial heart was created using two HeartAssistS VADswhere by one VAD pumps blood throughout the body and the other circulates blood to and from the lungs.
- HeartWare International announced in August 2009 that it had surpassed 50 implants of their Heartware Ventricular Assist System in their ADVANCE Clinical Trial, an FDA- approved IDE study. The study is to assess the system as bridge-to-transplantation system for patients with end -stage heart failure. The study, Evaluation of the HeartWare LVAD System for the Treatment of Advance Heart Failure, is a multicenter study that started in May 2009.

The majority of VADs on the market today are somewhat bulky. The smallest device approved by the FDA, the HeartMate II, weighs about 1 pound and measures 3inches This has proven particularly important for women and children for whom alternatives would have been too large.

One device gained CE Mark approval for use in the EU and began clinical trials in the US (VentrAssist). As of June 2007 these pumps had been implanted in over 100 patients.

Ventracor was placed into the hands of Administrators due to financial problems and was later that year liquidated. No other companies purchased the technology, so as a result the VentrAssist was essentially defunct. Around 30-50 patients worldwide remain supported on VentrAssist devices as of January 2010.

The Heartware HVAD works similarly to the VentrAssist- albeit much smaller and not requiring an abdominal pocket to be implanted into. The device has obtained CE Mark in Europe, and FDA approval the US. Recently it was showthat the HeartWare HVAD can be implanted through limited access without sternotomy.

In a small number of cases left ventricular assist devices, combined with drug therapy, have enabled the heart to recover sufficiently for the device to be able to be removed. HEARTMATE II LVAD pivotal study

A series involving the use of the HeartMate II LVAD have proven useful in establishing the the viability, and risks of using LVADs for bridge-to-transplantation and destination therapy.

- The pilot trial for the HeartMate II LVAS began in November 2003 and consisted of 46 study patients at 15 centers. Results included 11 patients supported for more than one year and three patients for more than two years.
- The HeartMate II pivotal trial began in 2005and included the evaluation of HeartMate II for two indications: Bridge to transplantation(BTT), and destination therapy(DT), or long-term, permanent support. Thoratec announced that this was the first time the FDA had approved a clinical trial to include both indications in one protocol
- A multicenter study in the United States from 2005 to 2007 with 113 patients (of which 100 reported principal outcomes) showed that significant improvements in function were prevalent after three months, and survival rate of 68% after twelve months.
- Based on one-year followup data from the first 194 patients enrolled in the trial, the FDA approved HeartMate II for bridge-to-transplantation. The trial provided clinical evidence of improved survival rates and quality of life for a broad range of patients.
- Eighteen- month followup data on 281 patients who had either reached the study end-point or completed 18 months of post-operative followup showed improved survival, less frequent adverse effects and greater reliability with continuous flow LVADs compared to pulsatile flow devices. Of the 281 patients, 157 patients had undergone transplant, 58patients were

continuingwith LVADs in their body and 7 patients had the LVAD removed because their heart recovered; the remaining 56 had died. The results showed that the NYHA class of the heart failure the patients had been designated had significantly improved after 6 months of LVAD support compared to the pre-LVAD baseline. Although this trial involved bridge-to-transplant indication the results provide early evidence that continuous flow LVADs have the advantage in terms of durability and reliability for patients receiving mechanical support for destination therapy.

- Following the FDA approval of HeartMate II LVAD for bridge-to transplantation purposes a post-approval (registry) study was undertaken to assess the efficacy of the device in a commercial setting. The study found that the device improved outcomes, both compared to other LVAD treatments and baseline patients. Specifically, HeartMate II patients showed lower creatinine levels, 30-day survival rates were considerably higher at 96% and 93% reached successful outcomes (transplant, cardiac recovery or long-term-LVAD).

HARPS

The Harefield Recovery Protocol Study (HARPS) is a clinical trial to evaluate whether advanced heart failure patients requiring VAD support can recover sufficient myocardial function to allow device removal (known as explantation). HARPS combines an LVAD (the HeartMate XVE) with conventional oral heart failure medications, followed by the novel B2 agonist clenbuterol. This opens the possibility that some advanced heart failure patients may forgo heart transplantation. To date, 73% (11 of 15) of patients who underwent the combination therapy regimen demonstrated sufficient recovery to allow explantation and avoid heart transplantation; freedom from recurrent heart failure in surviving patients was 100% and 89% at one and four years after explantation, respectively; average ejection fraction was 64% at 59 months after explantation- all patients were NYHA Class1; and no significant adverse effects were reported with clenbuterol therapy.

REMATCH

The REMATCH (Randomized Evaluation of Mechanical Assistance for the Treatment of Congestive Heart Failure) clinical trial began in May 1998 and ran through July2001 in 20 cardiac transplant centers around the USA. The trial was designed to compare long-term implantation of left ventricular assiat devices with optimal medical management for patients with end-stage heart failure who require but do not qualify to receive cardiac transplantation. As a result of the clinical outcomes, the device received FDA approval for both indications, in 2001 and 2003 respectively.

The trial demonstrated an 81% improvement in two-year survival among patients receiving HeartMate XVEcompared to optimal medical management. In addition, a destination therapy study following the REMATCH trial demonstrated an additional 17% improvement (61% vs 52%) in one year survival of patients that were implanted with a VAD (HeartMate XVE) with an implication for the appropriate selection of candidates and timing of VAD implantation.

A test carried out in2001 by Dr. Eric A Rose and REMATCH study group with patients with congestive heart failure that were ineligible for a transplant showed a survival at two years of 23% for those implanted with an LVAD compared with 8%for those who were treated with drugs. The two major complications of VAD implantation were infection and mechanical failure.

According to a retrospective cohort study comparing patients treated with a left ventricular assist device, versus inotrope therapy while awaiting heart transplantation, the group treated with LVAD had improved clinical and metabolic function at the time of transplant with better blood pressure, sodium-blood urea nitrogen and creatinine. After transplant, 57.7% of the inotrope group had renal failure versus 16.6% in the LVAD group; 31.6% of the inotrope group had right heart failure versus 5.6% in the LVAD group; and event- free survival was 15.8% in the inotrope group versus 55.6% in the LVAD group.

COMPLICATIONS AND SIDE EFFECTS

Early postoperative bleeding complications are a major cause of morbidity and reoperation in LVAD patients. Bleeding is the most common postoperative early complication after implantation or explantation of LVADs, necessitating reoperation in up to 60% of recipients. The implication of massive blood transfusions are great and include infection, pulmonary insufficiency, increased costs, right heart failure, allosensitization, and viral transmission, some of which can prove fatal or preclude transplantation. When bleeding occurs, it impacts the one year Kalan-Meier mortality.

In addition to complexity of the patient population and the complexity of these procedures contributing to bleeding the devices themselves may contribute to the severe coagulopathy that can ensue when these devices are implanted. Critical in the management of bleeding in the early hours after implantation or explantationis to adequately evacuate the post-surgical blood from around the heart and lungs to prevent retained blood from contributing to the need for reoperation to wash out clot that can compress the device features and contribute to post-operative shock. Preventing chest tube clogging during this period is critical to recovery. Because these devices result in blood flowing over a non-biologic surface, predisposing the blood to clotting, there is need for anticoagulation measures. One device, the HeartMate XVE, is designed with a biologic surface derived from fibrin and does not require long-term anticoagulation (except aspirin); unfortunately this biologic surface may also predispose the patient to infection through selective reduction of certain types of leukocytes. New VAD designs which are now approved for use in the European Community and are undergoing trials for FDA approval have all but eliminated mechanical failure.

VAD related infection can be caused by a large number of different organisms.

- Gram positive bacteria(Staphlococci, especially Staph Aureus, Enterrococci)
- Gram negative bacteria (Pseudomonas aeruginosa, Enterobacter species, Klebsiella species)

Fungi, especially Candida specie treatment of VAD- related infection is exceedingly difficult and many patients die of of infection despite optimal treatment. Initial treatment should be with broad spectrum antibiotics, but every effort must be made to obtain appropriate samples for culture.

Other problems include immunosuppression, clotting with resultant stroke, and bleeding secondary to anticoagulation. Some of the polyurethane components used in the devices cause a deletion of a subset of immune cells when blood comes in cotact with them. This predisposes the patient to fungal and some viral infections necessitating appropriate prophylactic therapy.

CHEST IMPLANTED LVAD

The Heart Ware Ventricular Assist System, a small left ventricular assist device that is implanted in the chest instead of the abdomen has been approved by the Food and Drug Administration as a bridge to heart transplant for the end-stage heart failure patients. The Heartware Ventricular System includes an implantable pump with an external driver and power source. The device is another treatment option for advanced heart failure patients, especially those who are smaller in size or can't have an abdominal implant. The approval of the continuous flow pump device comes less than 3 years after the agency approved Thoratec's HeartMate II left ventricular assist device (LVAD) for destination therapy. That device quickly replaced the previous generation of pulsatile devices. This is the first time that the FDA has approved a ventricular assist device using comparator data from a registry as a control, according to the agency.

The approval was based on data from the ADVANCE trial, which compared the outcomes of 137 patients implanted with the HeartWare System and of patients registered by the Interagency Registry for Mechanically Assisted Circulatory Support (INTERMACS). The registry has been in place since 2005. A total of 140 patients received the investigational pump and 499 patients received a commercially available pump implanted contemporaneously. At 180 days, 90.7% of the investigational pump patients and 90.1% of the of the controls had survived establishing the non-inferiority of the investigational pump. Induction right heart failure, device replacement, stroke, kidney dysfunction, hemolysis, and arrhythmia rates for the HVAD were similar to those reported previously for the HeartMate II.

Results of the ADVANCE trial showed that at 6 months, median 6-minute walk distance were improved by 128.5 meters and functional capacity and quality of life improved markedly and the adverse event profile was favorable. HeartWare registry data facilitated the development and availability of this new device. The registry is a joint effort involving the FDA, National Heart, Lung, and Blood Institute, Centers for Medicare and Medicaid Services (CMS), and clinicians, scientists, and industry. There is not enough data to show that the indications for VADs can be expanded to lower risk patients. Medicare currently does not have an open national coverage determination for VADs. Medicare currently reimburses VADs under certain criteria such as a bridge to transplant and as destination therapy. The 140 U.S. centers that place LVADs are expected to implant nearly 3000 devices this year. Nearly 4,600 patients have received an LVAD since 2010.

SYNCARDIA-TOTAL ARTIFICIAL HEART

The Syncardia Temporary Total Artificial Heart (Syncardia Systems Inc Tucson, Ariz) has now been implanted in more than 1,100 patients in approximately 100 centers in North America, Western Europe, Russia, Turkey, Israel, and Australia, this includes 125 implants, in 2012. It is a pneumonic biventricular, orthotopic pulsatile device that weighs 160 grams and displaces 400 ml. Blood flows through this device and follows a path that is nearly identical to the path through the normal heart. Flow rates in SynCardia patients are normally 7 to 9 liters a minute and there is very little turbulence within the device. The pneumatically activated diaphram system automatically balances blood output between left and right sides and also automatically responds to increased venous return with increased outputs. There is no suction.

To date the longest duration of support has been 3.75 years, in a man who has since survived after transplantation. More than 47 patients have survived for longer than 1 year of support and 72% of those underwent transplantation. In the bridge to transplantation, 70 to 80 per cent of patients have survived to transplantation even though they have been selected primarily from Interagency Registry for Mechanically Assisted Circulatory Support (INTERMACS) status 1(sickest patients) The survival rate for 1 year post-transplantation has been 80%to 86%. Most of the strokes associated with this device are immediately post-implantation (4%). Anticoagulation has included aspirin and warfarin in most centers. The stroke rate after the first two post-implant days in patients free of endo-device infection (98% are free)is 8 events per 100 patient years. Fatal infections associated with the device have been observed in 2% of the patients and spontaneous hemorrhage from arteriovenous malformations has not been observed. The survival rate to transplantation was 79%. A small group of patients sicker than usual were implanted during the study as "out of protocol compassionate use" patients with nearly 100% mortality rate.

Patient selection patterns that have focused on bridge-to-transplantation in adults may soon change. A destination-therapy application has been approved by the FDA and a smaller 50-ml pump is scheduled for use in smaller adults and children down to a weight of about 49 kg. A second generation <13-lb portable driver and an improved console are ready for widespread use. Dissemination of the Syncardia TAH-t has been hampered by lack of portable drivers and there have been only 36 "Big Blue" in-hospital drivers to support the entire world market. Hundreds of portable drivers are now available, and by 2014 the availability of small "in-hospital" drivers and portable drivers will no longer be restrictive.

Other trends noticed this past year,1)Nearly 20% of implants are for left ventricular assist device (LVAD) failure. 2) Increasing use has been noted for graft failure in cardiac transplant recipients. Graft failure is the major cause of death after cardiac transplantation. 3) Several centers once considered strogholds of an "LVAD-only" philosophy have become or applied to becoming Syncardia implanting Centers. 4)There is increasing use of the 70-ml device in pediatric cardiac surgical centers for congenital heart lesions.

Home discharge with total artificial heart

Home discharge with total artificial heart is feasible according to a report by Dr. Kasirajan of the Virginia Commonwealth University. Some patients with a total artificial heart can safely go home with the use of a small portable driver while awaiting heart transplantation. Researchers assessed 13 total artificial heart recipients who were stable enough clinically to be transitioned from the usual driver to SynCardia Systems investigational portable driver, The Freedom Driver System. The driver weighs 14 pounds and allows several hours of untethered activity. Eight of the patients were able to go home for an average of 5.5 months. They had a low rate major bleeding and no major infections. There were roughly five device malfunctions per patient year but in all cases patients were able to switch to a backup driver uneventfully. The Freedom driver is effective in supporting circulation with a total artificial heart. Discharge home was felt to be safe and feasible. Further data is expected to show the efficacy and safety of the driver. Important data on exercise capacity and quality of life will be valuable to moving the artificial heart technology to more widespread use. Dr. Dewey of Medical City Specialists in Dallas noted "The majority of patients on axial flow left ventricular assist devices are discharged home". He stated that they are sending close to 80% of patients home who are on total artificial heart. Dr. Kasirajan also noted that they have two patients at home for more than two years without readmission related to the device. One of the reasons that more patients on artificial hearts cannot go home is that the circulatory system has to be powered by compressed air. The new driver has two batteries that allow up to 3 hours of untethered activity. The ongoing study of the driver will enroll up to 60 patients from 30 international sites. Overall, 5 of the 13 current patients remained in the hospital (for medical reasons, discharge logistics, or personal preference) Where-as the remainder went home with the driver. The mean duration out of the hospital in the latter group was 162 days. The 13 patients had maintenance of cardiac function and their laboratory values remained stable. The five device malfunctions in the out of hospital were due to a valsalva maneuver, a faulty sensor, hypertension, a kink in the drive line, while the patient was getting into a car, and a driver dropped in the shower. All these patients remained stable and were able to switch to the backup driver as educated and returned to the hospital. Only a single patient in the out-of- hospital group died before transplantation. This patient was stable on the driver for 437days but experienced a fall with a spinal hematoma and developed fatal complications.

CHAPTER 13

Lung Surgery-Tuberculosis And Cancer

WHEN ONE THINKS thoracic surgery you automatically think of lung surgery that is resectional surgery for various pathological conditions such as tumor or infections or anatomical abnormalities such as bronchiectasis or emphysema. Cancer of the lung usually results in death if left untreated, the other conditions are associated with prolonged disability and may end in death or destruction of the lung tissue if left untreated. Both cancer of the lung and tuberculosis have been associated with milestones of surgical development and thus our discussion will center on these. Most of the major changes that we will discuss happened in the first half of the twentieth century for reasons that we have alluded to previously namely the development of antibiotics to control infection and the sophistication of anesthetic technique and agents.

Tuberculosis was the scourge of the population in the 19th century but with the advent of isoniazid, rifampin and streptomycin in the 20th century the death rate in the United States fell from 200 cases per year to less per year in 1980. The total number of new cases per year of mycobacterial infection in 1982 was 25,000. With modern antibacterial chemotherapy less than 2% will require surgical treatment. However there is an icreasing number of resistant TB bacilli and atypical TB bacillus. Historically Hippocrates wrote about phthisis as TB was called then. In 1839 Schonlein used the term tuberculosis and described the pathological changes. This disease spred quickly in Europe. The etiology of the disease remained obscure until Koch's description and isolation of the organism. By 1950 there were 100,000 sanatoria beds in the United States. Collapse therapy for pulmonary tuberculosis dates back to 1821 and was used as a surgical therapy sporadically in the last 20 years of the 19th century and during the first 50 years of the 20th century. Artificial pneumothorax and a variety of thoracoplasy techniques, principally rib resection were used during the first 50 years of the 20th century but not widely.

The first resection was performed by Block in 1882 however the patient died. It was not until 1936 that the first lobectomy and pneumonectomy for tuberculosis were first reported. Until chemotherapy became available in 1944 resectional surgery for tuberculosis carried a nearly prohibitive mortality. The 1950s and the 1960s were the important and most successful eras for the surgical treatment of tuberculosis.

The original isolation and staining techniques used by Koch are still good today. The mycobacterium(tuberculosis)that he isolated are still pertinent today and responsible for most clinically significant disease. Atypical bacterium as a group are often resistant to drugs and now represent about 50% of patients referred for surgery. Subgroups are described but not significant to the surgeon except to say they are resistant to drugs. Empiric five and six drug long-term chemotherapy when tolerated has achieved conversion to sputum negative status for patients with M. intracellulare disease. Localized pulmonary disease responds to excisional surgery combined with chemotherapy in well over 90% of these patients.

The pathology of tuberculosis of the lung (It may also infect other organs such as the kidney, the spinal cord) follows inhalation of the acid fast organisms. These tend to go to peripheral locations that cause an exudative alveolitis that progresses to caseous necrosis. The organisms get into the lymphatics resulting in enlarged lymph nodes of the hilum while the peripheral infection calcifies called the Ghon complex. This may be a quiescent lesion or there may be reactivation of the lesion as often seen in older or middle aged individuals. Direct progression of a primary lesion is most frequently seen in childhood. Post primary infection with progression is seen most often in apical and posterior segments of the upper lobes and the superior sections of the lower lobes This begins as an infiltrate and progresses to cavitation. Cavitation requires communication with the bronchial tree and thus spread throughout the lung. A fibrous reaction occurs around the lesion, acid fast bacilli are found, small cavities fuse into larger cavities and the segment, the lobe, or the entire lung is involved by the process with destruction of the organ that is hard to conceive until it seen as a specimen in the pathology lab. While this is a discussion of tuberculosis the pathology and destruction is similar to that found in many other mycotic diseases of the lungs such as blastomycoses, histoplasmosis, coccidiomycosis, and cryptomycosis. Endobronchial tuberculosis may result as the infection spreads causing swelling which may lead to obstruction and bronchiectasis of a segment or lobe and secondary infection by other micro organisms such as aspergillus. The organisms may involve the pleura with rupture of a bronchus that leads to empyema or a bronchopleural fistula. All in all not a pretty picture and one that usually requires some form of surgical intervention.

During the nineteenth century surgery for tuberculosis was limited to collapse therapy and thoracoplasty. It had been noticed that a coincident pneumothorax was sometimes associated with a remission of the disease. The concept of collapse of the upper lobes became a popular idea but results were often limited by plural adhesions. Even worse these attempts at collapse resulted in tuberculous empyema that required drainage and at times a thoracoplasty to close the cavity. A variety of other techniques were tried to collapse the upper lobes including unilateral phrenic nerve paralysis, separating the pleura from the chest wall and filling this space with paraffin, air fat, or other foreign bodies. This type of plombage thoracoplasty would bring about collapse of the upper lobes without interfering with the ventilation of the middle or lower lobes. Sputum conversion was achieved in 30 to 60 percent of patients. Another advantage was that it did not interfere with chest wall motion like a rib thoracoplasty would. From the beginning of the twentieth century until chemotherapy was available in the 1940s and 50s extrapleural paravertebral thoracoplasty was the most commonly used surgical procedural for the treatment of pulmonary tuberculosis. Without chemotherapy thoracoplasty achieved closure of cavities in more than 80% of patients with an operative mortality of approximately 10%. The development of chemotherapy in the 1940s made resectional surgery less hazardous though thoracoplasty is felt useful for bronchopleural fistulas and empyemas and sometimes for bronchopulmonary fistulas in other surgeries. Thoracoplasties cause an irreversible loss of ventilator capacity on the operated side.

The story of chemotherapy is important in two aspects 1) it made resectional surgery possible 2) it sharply reduced the number of patients requiring surgical treatment. And it made resectional surgery much safer. Block in 1882 performed excision of both apices of the lung for pulmonary tuberculosis on a relative who died postoperatively. Until 1940 attempted resections were performed by tourniquet and mass ligation technique and pneumonectomies had a 40% mortality whereas lobectomies perfomed up to that time had a 21% mortality and only 30% of survivers were well at the time of the report. In 1933 when the mortality rates from excision of the lobe of a lung was about 50% due to clumsy techniques and septic complications Edward d churchhill MD was able to show how to safely and selectively remove diseased parts of the lung.

That same year Evarts A Graham MD perfomed the first successful pneumonectomy for cancer of the lung on a 48 year old patient who survived for 30 years after the operation. However a description of his technique in that first resection showed the use of gross ligation and use of tourniquetes rather than the selective ligation of vessels and bronchi as described by Churchhill and and others such as Reinhoff, Blades and Kent and is used in modern operations. Effective chemotherapy with the discovery of streptomycin and PAS rapidly reduced the mortality and morbidity of resectional surgery of the lungs. By 1953 Chamberlain was able to report a series of 300 segmental resections for pulmonary tuberculosis with a 3% mortality and and a 93% cure rate. Resection replaced thoracoplasty as the common surgical treatment because it brought about conversion to sputum negative status in a single stage without deformity of the chest wall. A number of other drugs became available for use in tuberculosis that could be used by mouth or by intramuscular injection such as Isoniazid, Rifampin, Ethambutol, Pyrazinamide, Ethionamide, Para-aminosalicylic acid (PAS), Cycloserine, Kanamycin, and Capreomycin. The availability of these drugs have not only made surgery safer and more effective but has reduced the number of patients needing surgery leaving only the more complicated patients or those that did not respond to the drugs. More current reports indicate a mortality that can vary from 0% to 15%.

The most common cause of hemoptysis is tuberculosis. Identifying the site and source of the bleeding can be difficult and may even need to have immediate surgery. Bonchoscopy is done in the operating room to identify the lung and the lung may need or can be blocked with a cuffed tube before proceeding with the operation. The common source is a cavity. In children surgery is rarely used; ethambutol should not be used in the drug regimen. Bronchopleural fistula and empyema may occur and are difficult to treat. It should be first managed by tube thoracostomy however if it persists a surgical approach may be needed especially if there is recent excisional surgery.

LUNG CANCER

Lung cancer is the leading cause of cancer death in the United States affecting 200,000 individuals each year. It ranks first among males most often in the fifth and sixth decades and it is due primarily to cigarette smoking. The best treatment if possible is total extirpation preferably by a lobectomy or if necessary pneumonectomy. Small nodules may be removed by segmental resection but the findings have to allow for a complete resection though segmental resection is more useful for tuberculosis or nodules of unknown origin. Macewen of Glasgow is credited with the first pneumonectomy in multiple stages for tuberculosis. After removal of the left lung the pleural cavity was left open and packed it with gauze and later performed a thoracplasty. The first successful one stage pneumonectomy for carcinoma of the lung was performed by Graham in 1933. The technique of his first operation have been refined since then with a more sophisticated dissection at the time of surgery and less use of the disfiguring thoracoplasty. Auerbach and associates did a postmortem study of 117 males with multiple sections and convincingly showed the relationship of smoking and cancer of the lung. The combination of cigarette smoking and asbestos seems to be synergistic in producing carcinoma of the lung much like the stories of smokers in uranium or chromium mines. The fact that carcinoma of the lung can be produced using smoking dogs is another bit of convincing evidence of the relationship of smoking cigarettes and carcinoma.

The most common type is squamous cell carcinoma with an incidence varying from 40 to 70% of the total lesions. This type is associated with prolonged smoking of cigarettes. Squamous carcinoma is rarely seen in non smokers and in one series squamous cell carcinoma constituted only one% of the series. While squamous cell carcinoma usually spreds to distant organs it metastasizes less frequently to the brain and bones than does adenocarcinoma. Sqamous tumors tend to be large often with central necrosis.

Adeocarcinoma occurs in 5to 15% of the total and these tumors tend to be more at the periphery of the lung and more commonly in females. Adeno carcinoma has a tendency to metastasize to the liver, brain and bones.

Undifferentiated Carcinoma is present in 20 to 30% of the total and has often been termed as round cell or oat cell carcinoma.

Bronchiolar carcinoma is now recognized as a distinct type and is recognized to have a more favorable prognosis. In one series two/thirds of the patients had a resectable lesion with a 5 year survival of 48%.

In 1938, Friedrich described pulmonary carcinoma developing in scars secondary to other lung diseases and such changes have been recorded in scars of tuberculosis, trauma, infarcts, pneumoconiosis and other inflammatory disease.

Dual primary bronchogenic carcinomas have also been reported. The most common sites of metastases from carcinoma of the lung is the lymph nodes in the hilum and mediastinum. Clinical manifestations can vary from those that are asymptomatic to any variety of symptoms depending on their location, the location of metastases, even hormonal syndromes. Sometimes the lesion can be present for 5 or more years before producing symptoms. Common symptoms are cough, hemoptysis, chest pain, dyspnea, pleural effusion and clubbing. Other symptoms can include hoarseness, adrenal hyper-function, eosinophilia, liver enlargement, neuromyopathies, with sensory and motor loss, cortical and cerebellar plus psychiatric manefestations. Palpation of the cervical and axillary nodes often will indicate the progress of the tumor. The diagnosis will involve chest xrays, scanning films, broncoscopy, sputum cytology, and even percutaneous needle biopsy, and mediastinoscopy with a biopsy of hilar nodes and brain scan and bone scan and liver scan. The differential diagnoses will include pulmonary infection, pulmonary abcess, histoplasmosis, and rarely primary lymphosarcoma. Preoperative inoperability will include such signs as a bloody pleural effusion, Horner's syndrome, vocal cord paralysis, phrenic nerve paralysis, and superior vena caval syndrome. Radiation and /or chemotherapy is indicated for this last group

In those patients without evidence of distant metastases or local invasion in the chest surgical exploration is indicated. The operation in most cases will be a lobectomy though involvement beyond the lobe or involvement of mediastinum, pericardium or chest wall may require pneumonectomy along with nodal dissection or adjacent anatomy.

Video assisted thoracic surgery(VATS) is gaining prominence among phusicians who treat patients with Stage 1 or 2 non-small cell lung cancer and patients with a well defined pulmonary nodule. Vats lobectomy entails three incisions: a 2 cm camera port, a 2cm posterior port and a 4cm utility incision. No rib spreading is performed. Hilar structures are ligated individually, and mediastinal node dissection or sampling is performed under complete thorascopic visualization. Although several series were published over a period of roughly 8 years the number of patients were small usually 100 to 300 cases the most commonly cited series is one published by McKenna which involved 1,100 cases. In this series 9 deaths occurred (.8%) none of them introperatively or due to bleeding. Nine hundred thirty two patients (84.7%) experienced no postoperative complications. Blood transfusion was necessary in 45 patients(4.1%) and 28 cases (2.5%)were converted to thoracotomy. The median length of stay was 3 days and 180 patients(20%) were discharged on postoperative day 1 or 2. This attests to the benefits to the benefits of VATS lobectomy in properly selected patients.

DIAGNOSTIC THORACOSCOPY

Thoracoscopy refers to an examination of the pleural space or cavity with an endoscope. It originated in the hands of Hans Jacobaeus in Sweden in about 1910. The original reason for its use was to divide adhesions for lung collapse as a treatment in tuberculosis. Its use now is as a diagnostic tool rather than treatment. Fear of creating an empyema situation limited its use in the early years. Reports of Sattler in 1961 and of Berqvist and Nordinstam in 1966 and 1973 stimulated an interest again in the use of thoracoscopy as a diagnostic tool. A number of instruments that already exist are routinely used to perform thoracoscopy. The instruments available in most hospitals are fiberoptic mediastinescope, a rigid bronchoscope, a flexible bronchoscope, and a specially designed thoracoscope. Miniaturized endoscopes or special endoscopes have been developed for children. Local or general anesthesia are used though general anesthesia with an endotracheal tube is preferable to control ventilation and collapse of the lung. Lysis of adhesions may be appropriate for a thorough inspection which may reveal tumors, metastases, abcess, etc. This technique should not be used for empyema or in cases of proved lung cancer. A two trocar system can be used for insertion of a biopsy forceps if that is desired. This procedure usually follows bronchoscopy and mediastinoscopy using the same anesthesia. The patient is in the true lateral position.

THE TRACHEA AND ITS COMPLICATIONS

The trachea is the long cartilagenous tube that extends from the mouth through the neck and bifurcates in the mid-chest to provide the airway to the right and left lungs. The trachea has three distinct sections (1) the subglottic trachea which basically comprises the cricoid cartilage (2) the cervical trachea which extends from the first tracheal ring to the sternum (3) the mediastinal trachea which extends from the sternal notch to the carina and bifurcates into bronchi at the junction of the first and second parts of the sternum. At the top of this rather large tube composed of cartilaginous rings held together by flexible tissue is the larynx or the voice box that contains the vocal cords that provide the person with the ability to speak. The trachea and larynx are vital pathways for speech and breathing. It is obvious that anything that interferes with the passage of air to the lungs is life threatening. The laryngeal and cervical trachea is easily palpable in the neck which provides easy access if there is obstruction to air flow in the mouth or trachea and is easily accessible by a small incision in the lower neck with access to the lower trachea. In ordinary circumstances there is little of importance by way of vessels or organs and is an easy access to exposing the trachea for an incision and removal of a piece of two or three cartilages for insertion of a metal or plastic tube or a cuffed endotracheal tube through the tracheostomy if controlled ventilation is required. Upper airway obstruction can result from trauma to the mouth or neck, tumor, surgery, or even obstructing objects such as food, toys, vomiting and sometimes to control secretions in very ill patients. The trachea is kept distended by a series of C-shaped cartilaginous rings that are incomplete posteriorly in the so-called membranous portion of the trachea. These rings may be attached to each other lending some longitudinal stability. By extending the neck approximately half the of the trachea may be exposed by a cervical incision. And an additional length may be exposed and visualized by traction because the carina in the chest is mobile. Thus about two thirds of the trachea can be exposed by a cervical incision. The cricoid cartilage is a critical part of the anatomy because of the attachment of the vocal cords through the cricothyroid and the cricoarytenoid muscles. The recurrent or inferior laryngeal nerve which lies in a groove between the trachea and esophagus posterolaterly enters the larynx at the cricoid level and is closely related to the inferior thyroid artery. High tracheostomies involving the cricoid cartilage have a high incidence of subglottic stenosis and injury to the recurrent laryngeal nerve. Unlike primary diseases of the trachea, stenosis and malacia of the trachea secondary to postintubation injuries are common and are seen with increasing frequency. Cuffed tracheal tubes, long-term respiratory assistance and tracheostomy can produce a variety of tracheal wall injuries that heal as cicatricial strictures, as granulomas or as membranes. Tracheal malacia may be associated with these lesions at some point. Recognition of these possibilities and the importance of cuffed tube design has brought about a change in cuffed tubes and in the care and technique of tracheostomy and finally in the development of resectional surgery for the trachea. A nasotracheal cuffed tube at times is used for comfort if prolonged ventillatory assistance is required.

    The incidence of postintubation stenosis and malacia are difficult to obtain. However several studies such as those conducted by Grillo and Pearson and Andrews give us reasonable estimates of the relative incidence of clinical and sub-clinical stenosis. There are many cases of tracheal injury that heal with minor or moderate stenosis and deformity and do not pose clinical problems except perhaps under stress. The incidence of surgical obstruction requiring surgical correction is more evident. Grillo reported that the incidence of surgical obstruction in a vulnerable population of a respiratry unit was 17%. Pearson and Andrews reported a 20% incidence. Prospective studies indicate that the incidence of serious stenosis in patients undergoing prolonged respiratory assistance is 16 to 20%. The true incidence of surgical and non-surgical is much more difficult to define. Patients with an orifice of 5 mm or less have stridor at rest usually during inspiration. Mild and moderate strictures are usually not detected at rest. Though exercise may produce a wheeze or stridor. A brassy cough or difficulty raising sputum are consistent with milder forms of stricture. Gibson at the Royal Perth Hospital in Australia found a high incidence of tracheal ulceration and acute inflammation at the site of tracheal tube cuff (60%) at necropsies. However in the surviving patients 10 of 96 patients developed stenosis of varying severity and four of these required operation. Examination of the trachea in patients after intubation found significant changes at the tube site in every patient even in patients whose duration of the tube was as short as 1 day. The pattern of injury is ulceration healing and scarring though the degree of erosion and inflammation is related to the duration of use of the cuffed tube. Superficial tracheitis with fibrin deposits is seen in the first 48 hours. Ulceration of cartilages are seen in 3 to 7 days. Erosion into adjacent organs such as the esophagus or a blood vessel are known. These findings occurred in the era of high pressure cuffed tubes which has stimulated the use of low pressure tubes though even these changes have not eliminated superficial damage to cilia and mucosa. Significant surface damage may be produced in man and dog by low pressures and even uncuffed tubes. Surface morphplogy following uncuffed tubes reveals ciliary disorientation or ciliary denudation. Superficial infection is common and almost inevitable and may produce enough local destruction of the wall or its supporting cartilage to result in early or late stricture. Strictures related to the tracheostomy site are usually anterior. Tracheal stenosis was regarded as a rare complication until the production of cuffed tracheostomy tubes and their prolonged use for controlled and assisted ventilation. Early cases of tracheal stenosis occurred because of high tracheostomies involving the cricoid cartilage, the larynx, and the first ring of cartilage. In 1921 Jackson condemned the high tracheostomy because of a high incidence of laryngeal stenosis. There were few experiences with the problem until 1960 when the occurrence of tracheal stenosis after tracheostomy for respiratory assistance began to appear in the Belgian, French and American literature coinciding with the extensive use of cuffed tracheostomy tubes and ventilators. Large series of tracheostomies without prolonged ventilator assistance or cuffed tubes indicate that the incidence of tracheal stenosis is very low. Almost simultaneously with these reports there appeared reports of tracheal resection and end to end anastomosis. The strictures were the usual 2-cm long and 5-cm distal to the stoma. The excised tissue consisted of mature fibrous tissue without cartilaginous rings. Evidence that confirms the hazard of prolonged cuffed tubes was developed by Grillo and Shelley, Dawson and May in dogs with cuff pressures that varied from 35 to 214 torr. The lateral wall pressure could vary with the design of the of the tube especially the large volume, soft cuffed tubes where pressures could vary up to 100 or 200 torr instead of the more favorable range of 10 to 30 torr as in a modified Portex tube. Grillo found that the majority of patients developed symptoms from 10 to 42 days after extubation though the time interval could be short, a few days or it could be as long as 18 months. Rarely a granuloma at the tip of the tube may cause obstruction while the tube is still in place.

Tracheal stenosis usually manifests itself by stridor and difficult breathing. In milder cases it wll manifest itself at the time of severe exercise, difficulty clearing secretions, or a wheeze.

Definitive diagnosis can be made by laminograms of the trachea in anterior-posterior views, and lateral views. Most of the stenosis are just below the sternal notch and will not be seen on routine x-rays of the neck. Bonchoscopy is important to evaluate the presence and severity of the stenosis. A high or subglottic lesion may be seen on routine x-rays of the neck. The bronchoscopy is usually tolerated well so-long as dilatation or passage of the bronchoscope beyond the lesion is not attempted. There is a definite hazard of precipitating obstruction in the tight stenosis and perhaps the need to have a small bronchoscope or even a small tube available in case of precipitating obstruction either at the time of bronchoscopy or the delivery of anesthesia. A tracheostomy tube should be removed before taking x-rays though you should be prepared to replace it immediately.

Pulmonary functions are helpful indicaters for diagnosis. A slow inspiratory time is suggestive of a critical lesion. Vital capacity and forced expiratory volume of 1 second may be severely impaired. Vital capacity and forced expiratory time are impaired. Stridor at rest is usually associated with a lumen of less than 5 mm. The mild to moderate stricture without symptoms at rest are more difficult to identify. And these constitute about half of all strictures in a prospective study. These patients are often tagged and treated as having chronic bronchitis because of a brassy cough or a wheeze during exercise.

At surgery extension of the neck helps to bring the stenosis into view though the old tracheostomy may make dissection difficult. And the recurrent laryngeal nerves are avoided by staying close to the trachea. The principles of successful tracheal resection and reanastomosis are preservation of blood supply, avoidance of excessive tension and bacteriologic control. Circumferential dissection is avoided except at the site of stricture and one or two cartilages needed for the anastomoses. The trachea is freed from anterior tissue to the carina, this will avoid the inferior thyroid artery and the blood supply to the trachea that come posteriorly and laterally. Two to four cm of trachea is removed for the usual stricture. End to end anastomosis can be accomplished if no more than 4 cm of trachea is removed. The patient though should be warned about the possibility of a sternal splitting incision. Mobilization of the trachea down to the carina has increased the length of trachea that can be excised up to 5 or 6 cm. Laryngeal as well as hilar techniques will increase the length of resection that is possible. Prosthetic as well as natural tissue replacement have been worked on but there does not appear to be an ideal substitute for natural autologous trachea.

LUNG SURGERY

Lung surgery has a long and distinguished story. When one mentions thoracic surgery you automatically think lung surgery such as lobectomy and pneumonectmy for cancer of the lung. For the average thoracic surgeon who is not involved with heart surgery the lungs, the airways, the esophagus and the major vessels like the aorta and its branches become the primary focus of activity. The variety of problems that are encompassed by this part of thoracic surgery is large and we have touched on some of these as we progressed with our story

The 19th century witnessed a huge development of technical and diagnostic tools. We will review some of these though the first pneumonectomy for cancer was not performed until 1933.

The anatomy of the lung is essential to understanding the function and later surgical approaches to the pathology or malfunction. Malpighi in the 17th century demonstrated that the trachea terminated in dilated vesicles and that air passes in and out of vesicles. Malpighi also described the microscopic anatomy of the alveolus and described the pulmonary artery and veins. in 1880 Aeby and later Ewart, a pathologist described nine lobes and described 9 bronchial distributions. In 1932 Kramer and Glass established smaller units within the lobes which they termed bronchopulmonary segments. The importance of segmental anatomy was demonstrated by Churchhill and Belseys observation that patients with bronchiectasis of the left lower lobe also had involvement of the lower portion of the upper lobe which they termed the lingula. In 1943 the decisive studies of Jackson and Huber established the anatomical divisions that we use today. Basically the right lung has three major divisions or lobes and the left lung has two but each lobe has segmental divisions that have their own discreet blood and airway distribution. There are 12 pairs of ribs but only7 articulate with the sternum. There are 11 intercostal spaces between the ribs and these contain an artery, vein and nerve as well as muscle. The lining of chest cavity and the lungs is the pleura which can be divided according to what part it covers. The internal mammary artery and vein descends along the sternum to join the superior epigastric artery. The trachea is guarded by the larynx and descends into the chest and mediastinum to bifurcate into right and left branches that continue to branch to each segment and subsequently to each alveoli. It is covered by ciliated epithelial cells and a few goblet cells though the parts of the larynx that may come in contact with food and pressure are covered by epithelial cells. The terminal bronchiole divides into respiratory bronchioles then an alveolar duct and finally into the alveolar sac. The sacs open on all sides into alveoli which are now lined by epithelial cells. The alveolar epithelial sheet rests on a basement membrane that forms part of the air –blood barrier along with the basement membrane of adjacent capillary and its endothelium. Pulmonary capillary networks are the richest in the body. In emphysema there is destruction of the alveolar wall and supporting network. The pulmonary veins do not follow the course of the arteries.

Pulmonary lymphatic vessels enter the hilar region and ramify with plexiform channels along the bronchi and pulmonary arteries and veins. Pulmonary lymphatics do extend as far as the alveoli. The lymph nodes found along the lobar branches are called hilar nodes. There is a nerve supply that follow the vessels and airways to the lung. Right and left vagus nerves send one or more bronchial branches and a great many ganglion cells are found along the cervical and thoracic portions of the vagus nerves. There are collateral channels that form connections between well aerated alveoli and may serve as alternate channels if secretions are obstructive.

A knowledge of the gross and fine anatomy is helpful in interpreting the many diagnostic tools that are now available to the thoracic surgeon in the decision making process. Primary of course is the so-called routine chest xray which can point out gross abnormalities such as tumor, pneumonia, atelectasis, emphysema, pneumothorax, abnormalities of the chest wall and many other entities since the discovery of the x-ray by Roentgen in 1895.

With the localization of the pathology by xray, the development of endoscopy as a diagnostic technique, the rapid identification of bacterial and mycotic organisms and the development of anti- bacterial or antimycotic drugs the 20th century was set for the development thoracic surgery as we know it

CHAPTER 14

Robotics

ROBOTICS IS PERHAPS the newest addition to the developing field of mechanical and electronic aids for the surgeon and patient. General surgeons are rapidly adopting its use for laparoscopic surgery and it is also finding its place in thoracic surgery. One advantage is that it can give a three dimensional view of the critical field, another is that tremor is eliminated, and instruments can be angulated in any direction Thus it is used increasingly in place of laparoscopic surgery. It has its limitations but newer instruments are being added gradually such as cutting coagulation and stapling for larger vessels. There is a learning curve, laboratory training on animals is necessary and required and to some students may even be preferred bacuse it is 'easier' to do certain operations. The training obviously is a cooperatve effort of surgeons, institutions, and manufacturers. Safety and credentialing are obviously important considerations for the institutions that adopt It but more and more surgeons both general and thoracic are adding the use of this versatile instrument to their list of techniques. The most frequently used system today is the da Vinci Surgical System which is a multiarmed machine for complex endoscopic procedures. While it is a machine with many advantages for the general surgeon doing endoscopic surgery it is also finding a place in cardiac and general thoracic surgery. There are three arms to the instrument (1) the surgeons control handles, (2) the visual display (3) the user interphase panel. Another component is the patient's side cart wbich contains two or three arms that contain the operative instruments and one that controls video endoscope. Surgical robotics allow a surgeon to do coronary bypass anastomoses with limited incision and exposure. It allows surgeon now to implant valves at the bronchial segments orifice to treat some advanced and serious cases of chronic obstructive pulmonary emphysema particularly if they have already had stapling of diseased lobes or segments in their course of treatment so that air can get out but not get in. There are three bronchial current valves extensively studied. For instance there is the Emphasys EBV valve composed of a nitinol framework with a silicone sealant, a silicone one -way valve. Fine placement is achieved with the use of a broncoscope and a guide wire system. The umbrella-like device is passed down a bronchoscope and self-expands in the appropriate bronchus. There are numerous studies evaluating the Emphasys EBV. In one multicenter study 98 patients were treated by Reddy et al in India and Kaloo in the US using a pig model. Robotic procedures have been used in all forms of abdominal surgery e.g. splenectomy, cholesystectomy, Nissen fundoplication, and the technology allows for more complex procedures that could not be done with by standard endoscopy. Robot-assisted prostatectomies have been shown to be associated with reduced blood loss, and perhaps decreased incontinence and impotence.

The procedures emanating from this kind of orifice surgery are called Natural Orifice Transluminal Endoscopic Surgery. This new technology promises to become a useful technique in any part of the body with an orifice such as the lungs, the abdomen sexual organs and even the pleural space. Although there is a limited number of papers and experience with (notes) it may well prove a useful adjunct to lung volume reduction surgery by a reduction of non-functional lung along with improved stapling technique to reduce air leak.

CHAPTER 15

Mediastinum

THE MEDIASTINUM HAS its own list of problems. It has its own space and organs that provide a whole series of problems that are quite visible by routine chest films and very often definable by cat scans, mediastinoscopy, bronchoscopy, esophagoscopy and at times by palpation in the supraclavicular neck. It is the space between the pleural spaces. It has primary and secondary disorders. The most important of these are infections, emphysema, primary tumors and cysts. It contains the esophagus and major blood vessels such as the aorta the carotids and subclavian vessels and the trachea. We will deal with the esophagus and major blood vessels later as separate sections. Believe it or not the mediastinum has a history.

Prior to the introduction of endotracheal anesthesia few attempts were made to operate on mediastinal problems because of the fear of entering the pleural space. The Italian sugeon Bastianelli in 1893 performed one of the earliest operations removing a dermoid cyst fom the anterior mediastinum. Milton in 1897 devised a sternal splitting approach to the mediastinum that avoided the pleural spaces. He operated on a patient with caseating tuberculous nodes and even did a delayed closure of the sternum without difficulty 2 days later. The patient did well. With the introduction of the endotracheal tube for anesthesia which allowed the pleural space to be opened advances in the surgery of the mediastinum followed. Thoracotomy with intrapleural dissection is now the most common approach to the mediastinum but a sternal splitting incision is still used for anterior tumors or masses. The mediastinum is bound laterally by the mediastinal pleura and posteriorly by the vertebral column and anteriorly by the sterum. A plane extending from the lower manubrium to the fourth thoracic vertebra separates the superior from the inferior mediastinum. The inferior compartment is further subdivided by the pericardial sac into anterior, middle and posterior compartments. the superior mediastinum contains the trachea, the esophagus and the and the thymus gland. and the aortic arch and its branches. Located in the anterior mediastinum are the thymus gland and adipose, lymphatic and areolar tissue. The middle mediastinum contains the pericardium, heart, aorta, tracheal bifurcation, the main bronchi and the bronchial lymph nodes. The posterior mediastinum has the esophagus, descending aorta, and sympathetic and peripheral nerves. Acute mediastinitis is a serious condition which may be caused by perforation of the esophagus which may be caused by perforations during esophagoscopy, or a leaking anastomosis or tracheobronchial perforations as in bronchoscopy. High fever, tachycardia ad malaise and leukocytosis are common. There is usually severe pain in the neck and chest. The perforation of the esophagus is usually at the level of the cricopharyngeal muscle. Treatment requires drainage, antibiotics and eventually a surgical closure. Mediastinitis following cardiac surgery may be treated by debridement and reclosure of the sternum followed by continuous antibiotic irrigation. Chronic mediastinitis is usually due to a granulomatous inflammatory process such as tuberculosis or one of the other mycoses. Histoplasmosis commonly involves the lymph nodes of the mediastinum and is one of the agents responsible for mediastinal fibrosis. This may ultimately produce obstruction of the vena cava, the esophagus or the trachea. In one series of 7 patients with mediastinal fibrosis 4 patients required pneumonectomy. Because of the serious consequences of mediastinal fibrosis it is recommended that mediastinal granulomas be excised.

    The introduction of air into the mediastinum from anyone of numerous sources may produce a mediastinal emphysema. The source may be esophagus, tracheobronchial tree, a penetrating injury, trauma with fracture of ribs or vertebrae, even prolonged high pressure ventilation. The symptoms include substernal pain and crepitus in the lower neck. With increasing pressure the air may spread to the soft tissues of the chest, abdomen, and neck. In spontaneous mediastinal emphysema there may be a characteristic crunching sound that is synchronous with systole heard over the precordium along with subcutaneous emphysema in the neck. In this situation the emphysema usually subsides spontaneously. A common presentation with mediastinal emphysema is dysphagia. Recurrence of these episodes is uncommon. Chest films will show the air in the neck, pectoral muscles and occasionally in the extremities. Close observation, sedation, and administration are indicated and only rarely is surgery indicated.

Mediastinal Compression syndromes is most commonly due to penetrating wounds but also may be due to blunt trauma with transection of the aorta or other major vessels. Dissecting aneurysm are usually accompanied witth bleeding into the mediastinum. Following cardiac surgery especially following a sternal splitting incision and use of the hear-lung machine it is not uncommon to see an accumulation of blood in the mediastinum. Less common causes include anticoagulation, uremia, hemorrhagic diathesis, infection or bleeding from a primary tumor or cyst of the mediastinum. The spontaneous form of bleeding some times follow a violent form of coughing and with progressive bleeding mediastinal tamponade may occur with hypotension, cyanosis, dyspnea, venous distension and eccymoses at the base of the neck. Surgical treatment may be required to treat the source of bleeding and evacuate the blood. Obstruction of the superior vena cava may result from a variety of benign and malignant lesions involving the mediastinum. As the lesion progresses the symptoms are those of increased venous pressure such as edema of head, neck and upper extremities. This may be a progessive affair and the findings may become more prominent with the patient in the supine position. The majority of patients with superior vena caval syndrome have an underlying malignancy most commonly a bronchogenic carcinoma. Other malignancies include those of the thymus and thyroid. Of the 175 instances of superior vena caval syndrome 37 were due to mediastinal tumors, mostly lymphomas. In less than 1/ 4 of parients with superior vena caval syndrome the syndrome is the result of a benign process. Other causes include idiopathic mediastinal fibrosis, mediastinal granuloma (especially histoplasmosis) multinodular goiter, pleural calcification, and bronchogenic cyst.

Venous angiography will demonstrate the site of the obstruction. Surgical treatment is rarely indicated because the lesions are usually inoperable. Radiation treatment may produce symptomatic relief. Streptomycin infusion has been tried without success. Decompression of the superior vena cava may help at times using prosthetic or autografts but in patients with benign disease the process will improve spontaneously.

A large number of histologically different tumors and cysts may arise from the many structures located in the mediastinum. Since this site contains numerous lymph nodes metastases from other parts of the body are frequently found. Experience has shown that the majority of the primary lesions of the mediastinum can be cured by surgery and early diagnosis and surgical treatment is indicated. The neurogenic tumors are the most frequent neoplasms followed by thymomas, congenital cysts, and lymphomas. These frequencies turned up in a report of 1064 mediastinal tumors from a single institution. When tumor masses are found in the superior mediastinum the most likely diagnosis is thymoma or lymphoma. Tumors of the thyroid or para thyroid are less likely. There are exceptions such as the occasional neurogenic tumor may be found in the anterior mediastinum. As the tumor enlarges it will occupy more than one compartment of the mediastinum.

The most common medistinal neoplasms are the neurogenic tumors. These tumors occur at any age and are most often benign. In children these tumors have a greater tendency to be malignant. The list of neuorogenic tumors is long and includes such tumors neurolemmoma, neurofibroma, neurosarcomma pheochromocytoma and a few other variants. The 'dumbell" tumor may grow into the intervertebral space and thence into the spinal canal. CT scanning and myelography may be indicated if there is widening of the intervertebral space. There have been fatal complications when this condition was unsuspected. Neurogenic tumors other than pheochromocytosis may exhibit hormonal activity. Neurofibromas arise from nerve sheaths and nerve fibers of the posterior mediastinum. Two syndromes have been seen: diarrhea and abdominal distension; and hypertension, flushing and sweating. Ganglioneuromas arise from the sympathetic chain and and contain ganglion cells and nerve fibers. Ganglioneuroblastomas may behave in a benign manner if totally excised. Neuroblastoma is the general term for malignant tunors of the sympathetic system. These are highly invasive tumors most commonly seen in the retrperitoneal area in children but they also arise from any portion of the sympathetic system. These tumors generaly respond well to combinations of surgery, radiation and chemotherapy. One fourth of the patients did not respond favorably. Rare cases of spontaneous regression have been reported. A recently described syndrome of unknown etiology has been reported in 45 children with neuroblastoma, one half with mediastinal tumor. The condition described as opsomyoclonus, the "dancing eyes syndrome", is characterized by polymyoclonia, cerebellar ataxia, and opsoclonus and may be the first symptom of an occult neuroblastoma. These symptoms may disappear after resection but may also recur even without tumor. Nonchromafin paragangliomas usually arise from chemoreceptors and are usually adjacent to the aortic arch. These are almost always located in the paravertebral area The incidence of malignancy in paragangliomas and pheochromocytomas has been reported to be as high as 50%. The hormonally active tumors present with persistent or episodic hypertension. One report suggests that the middle mediastinum location may be more common. Extra-adrenal chromaffin tissue is present in branchial arch studies in coronary or aortopulmonary paraganglia, the autonomic tissue of the atria, or islands of tissue in the pericardium. The diagnosis of these tumors can be difficult using the standard items such as arteriography, venography, CT, and surgical exploration. Using enhanced CT with l-meta-iodbenzylguanidine scintigraphy the tumors were localized and surgically removed. Two or more of these tumors may be present simultaneously making diagnosis and surgical extirpation difficult.

Teratodermoid tumors are tumors composed of different types of tissue foreign to the area where they are found. These are an adult tumor. The solid teratoma differs from the dermoid cyst which belongs to this group and are usually found anteriorly in the mediastinum. These are very large tumors that compress adjacent tissue and sometimes rupture into the pleural space. Both endocrine and exocrine secretions have been documented from teratoid tumors. The occasional finding of inflammation surrounding tissue or bleeding have been ascribed to the secretion of digestive enzymes. Approximately 80% of these tumors are benign, there is poor correlation between size of tumor and age of patient. The newer classification of germ cell tumors and the relationship to tumor markers determined by radioimmunoassay and immune histochemistry has altered the current approach to patients with malignant teratomas. It is recommended that that patients suspected of having a malignant teratoma have measurement of tumor marker levels followed by needle biopsy to confirm the diagnosis. Combination chemotherapy including cisplatinum should be given followed by radical surgery after a fall of tumor markers to near normal levels.

THYMOMA Thymic lesions represent one of the most common types of mediastinal tumors. The association of thymic tumors with myasthenia gravis has long been known. These tumors usually appear in the anterior and superior mediastinum. They may be a small mass or or an ill-defined lobular mass and may located by CT scanning. The incidence of myasthenia gravis in patients with thymoma can vary from 10% to 50%. In one report 80% of patients older than 60 years with myasthenia gravis had a thymoma. The beneficial effect of thymectomy in patients with myasthenia gravis are well known. Myasthenia Gravis may occur with or without a thymoma. Thymomas may be benign or malignant though malignancy may be difficult to establish unless there are signs of invasion of adjacent organs or even distant metastases. Improved relief of symptoms are found with extended thymecomy rather than the limited form. It should be done with a sternal splitting incision. Thymomas have been associated with wide variety of conditions in addition to myasthenia gravis. There are reports that thymomas have been associated with red blood cell aplasia, Cushing syndrome, hypogammaglobulinemia, megaesophagus, and several collagen vascular disorders. The exact number of these are not delineated. Carcinoid tumors may be of thymic origin presumably arising from argentaffin cells within the thymus. Cysts may occur in the thymus and may be inflammatory, neoplastic or congenital.

LYMPHOMA

The lymph nodes of the mediastinum are frequently involved with disseminated lymphoma. Both Hodgkins diease as well as non-Hodgkins lymphoma may be present as primary tumors of the mediastinum though it is more likely that they are metastatic from a primary elsewhere. These tumors are characteristically in the anterior mediastinum although they may involve nodes elsewhere. Surgical excision followed by radiation therapy has been the standard however a combination of drug chemotherapy and radiation have produced a remarkable improvement in survival with both Hodgkins and non-Hodgkins lymphoma in the mediastinum. The operative goal is now limited to obtaining an accurate diagnosis.

PRIMARY EXTRGONADAL GERM CELL TUMORS OF THE MEDIASTINUM

These are not metastatic from the gonads but are from primordial mediastinal germ cells that did not complete their migration from the urogenital ridge. There are 5 types in pure or mixed forms. Seminoma, embryonal carcinoma, teratocarcioma, choriocarcinoma, and endodermal yolk sac tumors may be found. Considered together all germ cell tumors constitute 1-4% of all mediastinal tumors half of which are seminomas. Mesenchymal tumors found in the mediastinum include lipomas, liposarcomas, fibrosarcomas, myxomas, fibrous histiocytomas, tumors of muscle origin, and mesotheliomas. Treatment of these tumors is surgical. All are uncommon and have higher incidence in other parts of the body. These tumors show little response to chemotherapy or radiation. Vascular and lymphatic tumors are extremely common in other parts of the body but are distinctly uncommon in the mediastinum These tumors may be seen in all age groups and are found in any part of the mediastinum. These tumors can grow to large proportions before they are diagnosed and produce symptoms by compressing adjacent structures. Included with vascular tumors is the rare occurance of hematopoiectic tumors seen in association with spherocytic anemia. This mass is typically in the posterior mediastinum.

CYSTS OF THE MEDIIASTINUM

The cysts of the mediastinum form a significant portion of the primary lesions. Bronchogenic cysts originate from the ventral foregut that forms the the respiratory system and may occur in the lung or mediastinum. In the mediastinum they are usually located immediately posterior to the trachea or mainstem bronchi. A communication may exist with the tracheal lumen but usually they are adjacent to the trachea or have a cartilaginous attachment. Bronchogenic cysts are rare in infancy but when they do occur at an early age they may cause respiratory distress. In the older child they may cause severe respiratory distress by compressing the trachea or bronchus. CT scanning is useful in diagnosing these. They may compress the esophagus on barium swallow. In the rare patient with communication with the trachea a fluid level may be visible. Malignant degeneration has been reported.

ENTERIC CYSTS

Enteric cysts are also called enterogenous cysts, inclusion cysts, or gastric cysts these cysts originate from the dorsal division of the foregut. Duplications of the gut may be found at any level in the posterior mediastinum adjacent to the esophagus. They may be attached or embedded In the esophagus. Symptoms arise from pressure on the esophagus or trachea. Because these cysts are lined by gastric mucosa, acid secretion, ulceration, and bleeding are rcognized complications. The gastric mucosa allows them to be detected by technetium-99m scanning. A single case of adenocarcinoma has been reported. Enteric cysts are occasionally associated with vertebral anomalies and may be attached to the meninges or spinal cord.

PERICARDIAL CYSTS

These cysts are rather common mediastinal lesions usually occurring at the cardiophrenic angles especially on the right side. These are usually separate from the pericardial cavity though rarely communicate with it. These are rarely seen in children. Some patients have symptoms usually chest pain, cough and and dyspnea. This lesion is usually benign and the diagnosis is usually made from the routine chest film. The asymptomatic lesion is benign in 95% of the patients. In the syptomatic group there is a significant incidence of malignancy, in one report of 188 children with mediastinum tumors 72% were malignant. Symptoms that suggest direct invasion of nerves such as hoarseness, Horner's syndrome, and severe pain are generally associated with a poor prognosis. Since the incidence of malignancy is quite high surgical exploration is usually indicated. Some benign tumors may ultimately become malignant. The mortality accompanying these surgical exploration and removal of solitary tumors is negligible. Operations for myasthenia gravis has presented problems postoperatively but these respiratory problems clearly should be avoidable with modern assisted ventilation. Newer combinations of chemotherapy and radiation have improved survival for patients with Hodgkin's lymphoma, non Hodgkins lymphoma, but also for malignant thymoma, germ cell tumors and neuroblastoma. Sometimes there are late sequelae of the combined therapy such as pericarditis, coronary artery disease, pulmonary toxicity, scoliosis and even the development of another malignancy.

CHAPTER 16

Tumors Of The Esophagus

Esophageal Carcinoma

THIS IS ONE of the most feared and depressing malignant tumors. Its incidence is 5.7 per 100,000 white men and 20 per 100,000 per black men per year. It is more common in men than women though they tend to deveolop their cancers in the cervical esophagus or hypopharynx. There are variations of these statistics in other countries and cultures such as in Iran, South Africa, North China and even parts of Russia. The first successful esophagectomy was by Torek in 1913. Basically esophageal carcinoma is a disease of men in their sixth and seventh decades of life. But carcinomas of the hypopharynx and cervical esophagus occur in women almost as often and even more frequently in women as in men. This may be related to the greater incidence of Plummer -Vinson syndrome in women. (dysphagia with glossitis and atrophy of the mouth, tongue and upper esophagus). In Sri Lanka esophageal carcinoma is primarily a disease of women and is the most commonly encountered malignancy of the Gl tract. The etiology is unknown and many theories abound about food, hygiene, malnutrition, dental caries, vitamin deficiencies and even familial diseases and pre -malignant achalasia, reflux esophagitis, Barrett's esophagus, and leukoplakia. More than 95% of these carcinomas are squamous cell carcinomas. Adenocarcinomas arise either from the junctional columnar epithelium or the gastric cardia and rarely occur in the upper or mid esophagus. Barrett's Esophagus will be discussed later as a separate topic. In the Mayo Clinic experience with 1657 malignant esophageal tumors 8% occurred in the cervical esophagus, 25% in the upper esophagus, 17% in the mid esophagus, and 50% in the distal esophagus and cardia. This latter group may include a significant percentage of gastric tumors. It is generally accepted that squamous cell esophageal carcinoma occurs most frequently in the upper $2/3^{rd}$ of the thoracic esophagus, 2nd most frequently in the lower third and least commonly in the cervical esophagus. Other malignant tumors include (less than 1%) leiomyosarcomas, rhabdomyosarcomas, adenoacanthomas, carcinosarcomas, and primary malignant melanomas. Hematogenous and lymphatic spread are common and typically penetrate the entire wall of the vessel and invades contiguous tissue. Thus upper and middle third tumors tend to invade the tracheobronchial tree, aorta, and recurrent laryngeal nerve. Whereas the lower third tumors tend to invade the diaphragm, pericardium, or stomach. The extensive mediastinal lymphatic drainage which communicates with cervical and abdominal collaterals is responsible for the finding of mediastinal, supraclavicular, or celiac lymph node metastases in at least 75% of the patients with esophageal carcinoma. Lymph node metastases tend not to be segmental in distribution and spread to jugular, intrthoracic, or intra-abdominal nodes occurs with primary tumors located at any level.

Symptoms from esophageal cancers may be insidious and non-specific beginning with retrosternal discomfort. As the tumor enlarges the dysphagia becomes progressive with weight loss, chest pain and occasionally with hematemesis. Any patient who complains of progressive dysphagia needs a barium esophagogram and an esophagoscopy. Biopsy and washings will establish a diagnosis in over 90% of the time. Air contrast radiographic techniques are particularly helpful for small lesions. Benign smoothly tapered lesions by radiography still require esophagoscopy and biopsy. Most benign peptic strictures can be dilated with intraoperative forceful maneuvers or by postoperative rubber dilators of varying size that can be passed through the mouth into the esophagus with the help of local anesthesia. If an additional treatment is needed and the benign stricture is in the esophago-gastric area an anti-reflux procedure can be performed by several different procedures including the use of limited access techniques.

Once the diagnosis of cancer of the esophagus is made therapy may include surgery, radiation and/or chemotherapy. The results with either one alone have not been successful and therapy with a combination of one or two of these modalities will depend on the extent of the disease as judged by catscan or other radiographic procedures or biopsy of mediastinal nodes using mediastinoscopy (procedure from the neck) or even a limited evaluation through a small parasternal incision. Despite the fact that aquamous carcinoma is usually sensitive to radiation therapy, radiation alone seldom achieves cure. Radiation is usually used as an adjunct to esophagectomy. Approximately one half of the patients receives palliative course of 4000 to 5000 rads over a 4 or 5 week period. Even super voltage treatment of 5000 to 7000 rads has not achieved 5 year survival better than 10 to 20%. Results with either surgery or radiation it seems is less than 10%. That makes this a very deadly tumor. The surgery for carcinoma of the esophagus is usually thwarted by extensive spread beyond the visible bounds of the tumor. More than 80% of the patients die within one year. The Japanese have reported survival rates of 25 to 37.5% using preoperative radiation plus surgery. These results have not been duplicated in this country and there is some doubt about whether it is the same tumor. The operation for those in whom it offers the possibility of cure or salvage palliation will vary with the location of the tumor and usually involves resection of half or the whole esopgagus with substitute replacement by using (pulling up) the stomach or a long piece of the large colon for anastomosis to the remnant of esophagus in the chest or in the neck. This is a complicated operation of significant proportions usually done as a thoracic operation but may be done by incisions in the neck for the upper anastomosis and an incision in the abdomen to prepare the segment of colon or the stomach after removal of the entire esophagus. This is a dreaded diagnosis with limited chances of 5 year cure

Palliative intubation of esophageal carcinoma is available and offers a means of maintaining nutrition in those patients with total or near total obstruction. There are a number of tubes designed for placement through the area of obstruction so that there is a passage way for saliva and food or drink. These tubes are of two types pulsion tubes are for passage from above and pushed through the tumor with the aid of an esophagoscope and traction types which are pulled into place by downward traction through a gastrostomy (opening made in the stomach) made through a small opening in the abdominal wall. The average survival after palliative intubation is less than 6 months. This type of therapy is best suited to patients with trachea-esophageal fistula in whom an intraesophageal tube may both occlude the esophageal side of the fistula and permits oral alimentation for the remaining months of life. Such palliative bypass for incurable malignancies of the gastrointestinal tract have been applied to tumors of the stomach, biliary tract, panceas, and large and small bowel. The mortality rate for colon bypass of esophageal carcinoma is at least 15 to 25%. A number of other forms of gastric or colonic bypass for inoperable cancer of the esophagus have been advocated but all have a high mortality or complication rate as well as mortality rate.

Perforation of the Esophagus

Spontaneous rupture of the esophagus and instrumental rupture of the esophagus usually by an esophagoscope or some other instrument that is being used for therapy can produce life threatening or complication threatening situations. The first spontaneous rupture of the esophagus was reported by Boerhaave in 1704 in the Netherlands. Van Swieten gave an English version of the Boerhaave Syndrome "The illustrious Baron Wassenaer, Lord High admiral to the Republick, after intense straining in vomiting broke asunder the tube of the esophagus near the diaphragm, so that after the most excruciating pains the aliments which he swallowed passed together with air into the cavity of the thorax and he expired in 24 hours." Spontaneous or instrumental rupture are unusual. The absence of a serosal layer of tissue in the esophagus unlike the remainder of the Gl tract make it more prone to rupture at lower pressures. Ruptures of the lower esophagus almost always perforate into the left thoracic cavity and ruptures of the mid esophagus rupture into the right thoracic cavity. Swallowing a large bolus or vomiting rapidly enlarges the diameter momentarily up to 5x the normal diameter. Among the causes of esophageal rupture in addition to those mentioned is a swallowed foreign body, blunt chest or abdominal injury, acid-peptic ulceration, and penetrating missile. Rupture of the esophagus may result from primary esophageal disease or penetration by some missile. Death may occur within 24 hours. Early collapse of the patient is common. Chest pain, nausea, vomiting are common. Pain at the level of the perforation is common. When a strain induced tear is below the cardia bleeding rather than perforation is the dominant feature. In special circumstances patients have survived perforation of the esophagus. However surgical treatment is usually required. The operative approach depends on the cause and site of the perforation whether it be cervical or thoracic and the time elapsed following the perforation. Feeding is eliminated and intensive antibiotic therapy is started. Drainage and closure if it is in the neck. Alternatively an esophagostomy tube can be placed for drainage and feeding. In the thorax survival will depend on the time interval. Less than 24 hours the mortality may be 10-15%. If later the mortality will increase to 50%. The procedure will vary with the underlying problem. If it is a carcinoma a resection will be needed, myotomy in case of stricture, hiatal hernia repair with antireflux procedure in case of patients with reflux esophagitis. Simple closure of the opening will not solve the problem if there is an obstructing lesion below. Following surgical treatment continuing infection is a serious threat. Mediastinitis, empyema, abcess, and breakdown of the closure itself remain as serious potential problems and contribute to the high mortality. Restoration of adequate nutrition becomes important to survival.

CHAPTER 17

Barrett's Esophagus

THERE IS AN incidence of adenocarcinoma in Barrett's esophagus. In 1950 Barrett described a condition in which gastric epithelium lining the esophagus was usually associated with either ulceration in the gastric epithelium or esophagitis in the squamous epithelium proximal to the junction with abnormal mucosa. The cause of this is still undetermined. In a few patients it appears to be of congenital origin. However most patients with this condition have severe chronic longstanding reflux. Barrett's columnar epithelium may migrate proximally. It appears that columnar epithelium is capable of repopulating the denuded the denuded esophageal lining at the junction where the squamous epithelium is eroded by reflux of acid. A stricture of severe esophagitis frequently occurs at the junction of squamous and columnar epithelium. The columnar epithelium has been observed to undergo dysplasia or neoplastic change and a number of patients with adenocarcinoma of the esophagus are seen in whom the cancer seems to arise in the columnar epithelium. Multiple biopsies are recommended to rule out neoplastic change. If high grade dysplasia or neoplasia are found an esophageal resection should be performed. When only chronic reflux is diagnosed an antireflux repair should be performed following dilatation of any stricture that may be present. In most patients long term followup and repeat esophagoscopy are indicated if carcinoma is not found. The incidence of carcinoma seems variable and probably low. A study published in the New England Journal of medicine in 2012 by Dr. Frederik Hvid-Jensen of the department of surgical gastroenterology at Aarhus(Denmark) University and his associates reported that the incidence of esophageal adenocarcinoma with Barrett's esophagus was only 1.2 cases per 1000 person-years in a study of the entire population of Denmark. That rate is four to five times lower than rates reported previously. Their conclusion was that the risk of adenocarcinoma among patients with Barrett's esophagus is so minor that in the absence of dysplasia routine surveillance of such patients is of doubtful value. Most patients with adenocarcinoma of the esophagus do not have a previous diagnosis of Barrett's esophagus. A total of 11,028 patients underwent endoscopic biopsy and received a diagnosis of Barrett's esophagus. During 1992-2009, the median age was 63 years and patients were followed for 5.2 years. During that time, 197 of these patients with Barrett's developed new esophageal adenocarcinomas, which comprised 7.6% of all the 2,602 incident esophageal adenocarcinomas diagnosed in the general Danish population during 1992- 2009. The annual risk of developing malignancy was only. 12% or 1 case of adenocarcinoma per 860 patient years. In contrast reviews of the literature published in past decade in the United States and Europe calculated the incidence of esophageal adenocarcinoma as ranging from 5.2 to 7.0 cases per 1000 person years. A recent population based study based in Northern Ireland found remarkably similar results, an incidence of 1.3cases of esophageal adenocarcinoma per 1000 patient years among people with Barrett's esophagus supporting the conclusion of Dr Frederik Hvid-Jensen.

AORTA

The is one of those commanding blood vessels of the body that is key to life and is also subject to some of the most threatening complications that confronts a thoracic surgeon. It is the main vessel exiting the heart after it receives all the oxygenated blood from the lungs and branches to the whole body. It presents with anatomic anomalies in infancy as well as life threatening abnormalities such as aneurysmal dilatation in the adult especially in the elder population either from trauma or arteriosclerotic degeneration or inherited connective tissue weakness such as in Marfan's syndrome.

The first accurate description was by Galen in the second century. Fernelius in 1542 observed that aneurysms developed from a localized thinning of the arterial wall. Vesalius is credited with making the first accurate clinical diagnosis in 1557. Historically a number of attempts were made to treat aneurysms of the aorta. In 1785 John Hunter operated on a patient with an aneurysm and ligated the artery high enough above it to allow for one or two branches below it. Electrical stimulation to promote clotting was introduced by Benjamin Phillips in 1838. Another method of treatment was perchloride of iron presumably to induce clotting but this was not successful. Moore of London thredded 26yds of fine wire into one and Corradi passed a galvanic current through an aneurysm. None of these imaginative treatments succeeded. Matas in 1888 introduced endoaneurysmoraphy. He was the first to realize the importance of re-establishing the continuity of the vessel lumen. He devised three types of operations. One was restorative which was used for saccular aneurysms; one was reconstructive which made a new vessel out of the wall of the old vessel and finally the obliterative for fusiform aneurysms. He could rarely restore the lumen. In 1902 Tuffier operated on a patient with a saccular aneurysm of the ascending aorta. He applied two catgut sutures just distal to its neck but he did not excise it but it too failed because of necrosis caused by the sutures. There followed a host of attempts repeating the failures described above. Next followed attempts (1912) using wire and electrification. There were attempts of using cellophane to stimulate periarterial fibrosis. There were other attempts by Yeager and Cowley using dicetylphosphate in 1948 to stimulate periarterial fibrosis. None of these attempts yielded a satisfactory solution and mortality was significant. Here we are at the middle of the 20th century and no satisfactory technique for treating aneurysms of the aorta whether thoracic or abdominal. Matas in 1940 reported a cure that might have been the first cure of an abdominal aneurysm though the technique used would not be applicable generally nor acceptable today. It was a patient operated upon in 1924. He had ligated the aorta just above the large aneurysm with two half inch cotton tapes. For the first nine days the aorta was totally occluded and her condition was precarious. The ligatures yielded or relaxed and allowed some blood to flow. Collateral circulation was established both above and below the ligatures. Her death was due to tuberculosis. The aneurysm had solidified and lost all characteristics of an aneurysm. In 1940 Bigger and Elkin reported success in ligating an aneurysm. Bigger said that there had seen eighteen instances of ligation of the abdominal aorta since Astley Cooper did it in 1817 and six of these were successful. The first instance of resection of a saccular aneurysm of the aorta was by Byron and Alexander in 1941 in a boy of 19. At thoracotomy a diagnosis of coarctation was made on the basis of extrinsic pressure by a neoplasm. A diagnosis of a saccular aneurysm was made. Greatly enlarged blood vessels were noted both above and below the saccular aneurysm. The collateral circulation was strong with greatly enlarged vessels such as the intercostals and the subclavian. Cotton tapes were used to ligate the aneurysm above and below the aneurysm and the sac was excised. The ends of the aorta were oversewn with silk. Intercostals arising from the sac were ligated. When the aneurysm was removed his blood pressure rose to 250 over 130.

Postoperatively he had acute cardiac decompensation which responded to treatment and he was discharged with a blood pressure of 215/105. He later died of cerebral hemorrhage. In 1944 Ochsner resected a thoracic aortic aneurysm with success. At operation instead of tumor he found a small sacciform aneurysm of the descending aorta The base of the aneurysm was clamped and the aneurysm excised the wall of the aorta closed. She made an uneventful recovery. Monad in 1948 reported a similar case. In 1948 Cooley and DeBakey operated on a man for an aneurysm of the anterior superior border of the arch of the aorta. The base of the aneurysm was located between the innominate and the left common carotid. A no 24 french catheter was used to ligate the base of the sac. He had complete relief of pain and was discharged. Two months later he was readmitted to the hospital and died within 30 hours of hemorrhage. The mistake was in not excising the sac much as happened to tuffier fifty years before. In January, 1950 Cooley and DeBakey operated on a man for coarctation of the aorta. He also had a non-pulsating mass in the right supraclavicular region. Four months after the operation he was readmitted to the hospital because he had developed a recurrent laryngeal paralysis on the right and a partial right phrenic paralysis. He was operated on again with a diagnosis of aneurysm of the right subclavian which was 12x8 cm in size. The superior vena cava was obstructed and the right innominate vein and azygos vein were enlarged. The aneurysm was excised after ligation of the subclavian artery proximally and distally. He made an uneventful recovery. The first successful resection of an abdominal aortic aneurysm was that of dubost of Paris in 1951. The patient was a 50 year old man with a large mass in his abdomen. The aneurysm extended from the renal arteries to the iliacs. A clamp was applied to the aorta above the aneurysm just below the renal arteries and the common iliacs were clamped and sectioned. A 15 cm graft taken from a 20 year old women three weeks previously was put in place and sutured to the aorta and the iliacs with 5-0 silk. Not having a Y shaped graft the graft was first sutured to the right common iliac then the left iliac was sutured to the side of the graft. The patient made an uneventful recovery and was in good condition 5 months after. This is the first successful graft and anatomic restoration of the anatomy that provided a blueprint of future excision of aneurysms with anatomic restoration of circulation. The 1950s were years of significant advancement in heart surgery and the vascular surgery of the great vessels. In 1952 Johnson, Kirby and and Horn reported on the fate of homografts in pigs. The grafts were preserved in a nutrient solution and implanted in young pigs. Degenerative changes occurred in all. In 1953 Cooley and DeBakey again discussed the treatment of aneurysms and reported the first successful resection and graft replacement of a thoracic aortic aneurysm which was huge and had produced erosion of adjacent vertebral bodies. Bahnson in 1953 reported twelve successful resections, six thoracic and six abdominal. He replaced five of the abdominal aneurysms with homografts. In one he excised the aneurysm and sutured the wall. In 1955 Shumacker reported the surgical treatment of five cases of ruptured aortas with recovery in three. He used plastic grafts. He also collected 35 treated cases from the literature twenty- one had recovered (60%) and and 14 (40%) had died. In 1955, Johnson and Kirby and Lehr reported their experience using a glass tube much as Alexis Carrell had done back in 1910. They used this technique in two cases with success. In each case the aorta was occluded for only six to eight minutes. This is impressive as a technique but appears to be only an isolated experience. The direction of aortic replacement was clearly in the direction of graft replacement after cross-clamping the aorta. Hufnagel who was one of the first to use arterial grafts wrote about the use of rigid and flexible plastic prostheses for arterial replacement. He found orlon tubes to be successful in animals and used them in 15 patients with success. In 1950 Clatsworthy reported the use of siliconized polyethylene tubes as external shunts.

They showed a marked improvement in mortality and morbidity when the shunts were used. Shaferand Hardin in 1952 reported similar results but lost two patients with aneurysms of the aortic arch and of the aorta. but succeeded in the case of a vena cava –aortic aneurysm. In the same year Izant, Hubay and Holden were able to shunt 80% of the aortic flow through a large polyethylene tube. Cross, Kay, Jones and reported experimental work in which they shunted the left ventricle by way of the auricle to the aorta. In 1950 Clatsworthy reported the use of siliconized polyethylene tubes as external shunts and showed a marked improvement in mortality and morbidity figures when the shunts were used. In 1956 chamberlain and associates describe the case of a man of 63 who had multiple aneurysms of the aorta. They used two 25cm segments of a pigs aorta sutured together and used as an external shunt. The three aneurysms were resected and a 20 cm homograph was sutured in place to bridge the resection. The shunt was in place for two hours and 45 minutes. He did have a temporary memory loss and a recurrent laryngeal paralysis but left the hospital in good condition. In a discussion of this case Sewell said he had used a three limb shunt for division of the aorta proximal to the innominate artery. Bahnson reported a case in which he had used a shunt of homograft and resected the arch of the aorta. He was able to preserve the part of the arch from which the vessels to the head arose. Mahorner and Spencer described this technique in 1954. Dodrill said he had used shunts between the subclavian and the femoral arteries. Bahnson and Nelson in 1956 wrote about cystic medial necrosis as a cause of localized aortic aneurysms amenable to surgical treatment. They had operated on 5 patients with complete recovery in two, temporary recovery in one, and postoperative deaths in two. They said that Erdheim's cystic medionecrosis was often present in dissecting aneurysms and was thought to be the chief cause of the dissection in young individuals. This necrosis was thought to be the cause of spontaneous rupture. It is also a chief feature of Marfan's syndrome. When the ascending aorta is involved the aortic valve may be incompetent. Histologically lesions consist of necrosis and disappearance of muscle cells and elastic laminae. The first description of the pathology was made by Gesell in 1928.

For some two or more centuries examples of traumatic aneurysms have been recorded. In 1947 Strassman collected 72 cases from the literature. Forty were at a point just distal to the ligamentum arteriosum and fourteen were in the ascending aorta just beyond the valves and the remaininder were in the descending and abdominal aorta. In only three cases could he record traumatic rupture of the abdominal aorta. Diagnosis is not easy and symptoms maybe entirely absent. Widening of the mediastinal shadow is a characteristic finding. If there is doubt angiocardiography should make the diagnosis.

The first successful case was that of Bahnson in 1952. In 1956 and 1957 when he did an aneurysmoraphy, eleven cases with 2 deaths. Gerbode operated on four using a pump-oxygenator. Cooley in l956 used the pump-oxygenator on a traumatic aneurysm with success. Storey, Nardi and Sewell reported two cases with successful resection and graft in one case. In 1956 Cooley and DeBakey reported on their success resecting the entire ascending aorta because of a fusiform aneurysm with the aid of the pump-oxygenator. In 1956 DeBakey and Cooley reported on their experience with aortic aneurysms. They had operated on three hundred and thirteen cases. Eighty- three were thoracic and two hundred and thirty were abdominal. There were 24 saccular aneurysms and excisions were done with reconstruction of the aortic wall and nine deaths. There were forty three fusiform aneurysms of the thoracic aorta and fourteen deaths (33%). There were sixteen dissecting aneurysms with 3 deaths (19%); two hundred and thirty abdominal aneurysms with rupture in 27 and 9 deaths (3.9%); unruptured in 203 with 17 deaths (8%). A total of fifty-two deaths among three hundred and thirteen cases (17%). Six had extensive thoracoabdominal aneurysms which required the use of a temporary shunt for its resection. In treating dissecting aneurysms they divided the aorta and sutured the rims to close off the dissection. This represented a marked decline in mortality. In 1952 the mortality was 25%; in 1956 it was down to 2%. One third of all deaths occurred as a result of acute rupture. In 1957, Schimert, Hadrian and Bratigan reported a case of a fifty-one year old who had an aneurysm of the arch of the aorta. They used a temporary bypass of the area for 45 minutes while the arch was resected and replaced with a homograph.

The subject of homograft vs artificial or plastic grafts was covered by a committee of the society for vascular surgery in 1957. They had decided that synthetic grafts could be used effectively. They reported a 93% success in 256 cases. DeBakey said that he knew of over a thousand cases of diseases and injuries of the aorta which had been operated on. Grafting had been used in 80%. Homografts had been used in 84% of these and plastics in 16%. Among one hundred and eleven in which the Orion or Edwards Tapp type had been used the incidence of complications had been low and predicted that the artificial or plastic grafts would eventually replace the homografts. The most satisfactory materials were Dacron and Teflon. Sanger, Taylor, Matsuba and Salmone reported on their use of Knitted, seamless Orion and Nylon tubes as arterial grafts and showed in dogs that a fibrous layer both inside and outside the graft with a growth of tissue through the interstices of the graft. They said that 24 surgeons had used the seamless Knitted Orion grafts in78 patients with success. Edwards and Tapp used a new braided Y tube of nylon treated chemically with formic acid to bypass the aortic bifurcation obstruction in four cases with success. Kirklin and his associates reported their experience in the surgical treatment of thoracic aortic aneurysms. They had operated on 20 but had been able to resect only fifteen. Grafts were used in all but one in which excision and lateral suture of the aortic wall was possible. They used homografts in all but two in which they used ivalon. The aorta can be safely cross clamped for eighteen to forty five minutes. Hypothermia was used in all at less than 30 degrees and it was estimated the that at that temperature it was safe to cross clamp for up to an hour. The arterial homograft remains functionally and structurally adapted to its new environment and fuction and is not replaced by other tissue. The last word on synthetic grafts for the aorta from Crawford, DeBakey and Cooley in 1958 who reported the use of synthetic grafts in 317 cases. In 210 cases they had used Dacron knit tubes and the circulation had been restored in 98% of the cases. Using Orion knit and Nylon-Dacron knit tubes the results were 94% successful. These are somewhat rigid and resist the passage of a needle. Usng Edwards tapps tubes they had success in93%. They used Orion taffeta tubes in 13 with success in 86%. Ivalon sponge tubes were used in twelve patients and were successful in only 42%. Studies on plastic tubes in dogs show tha Dacron, Orion and Teflon maintained most of their strength during the period of observation but only Teflon showed absence of complications.

DISSECTING ANEURYSM OF THE AORTA

The first description of a dissecting aneurysm of the aorta was given by Laennec in 1830. He described the dissection of the intima by an enlarging hematoma. DeBakey pointed out that it is rapidly fatal in over 75% of the cases. Burchetl in 1955 said that it was almost always associated with hypertension. In 1934 Shennan made a study of two hundred and eighteen cases and decided that atherosclerosis was not an important factor. Most frequently rupture occurs in the arch of the aorta, usually not far from the aortic valve. Schnitker and Bayer made the observation that 50% of their women with dissecting aneurysm were pregnant. Characteristically there is a history of severe pain which usually radiates posteriorly in either the thoracic or lumbar regions. Also the pain usually advances caudad from the thorax to the back of the abdomen and finally to the extremities. The condition may be confused with a myocardial infarction. The x-ray of the chest is important because it shows a mediastinal widening of the shadow involving the thoracic aorta. Golden and Weens showed that angiocardiogram is the most valuable tool for making the diagnosis. Schnitker and Bayer in 1944 did a study of dissecting aneuycm in young people. They found a record of 580 cases in the literature with 24.3% under the age of 40 whereas coronary arterial disease occurs in only 1.54% of this age group. Glendy, Levine and White found one hundred and forty one cases in people under forty and of these forty nine were females with pregnancy in twenty-four. The first attempt to correct this condition surgically was made by Gurin, Bulmer and Deby in 1935. They exposed the bifurcation of the aorta and opened one of the iliacs which revealed the double barrel lumen and they excised a portion of the intima to make a reentrant site. The previously pulsations reappeared in the dorsalis pedis artery but the patient died on the sixth postoperative day. The first successful repair of this condition was reported by DeBakey, Cooley and Creech in 1955. They pointed out that in the patints who survived the acute dissection there is some point of re-entry rupture where the false lumen again communicates with the true lunen. They operated on six patients and four recovered. After cross clamping the aorta they transsected it noting the double lumen. They sutured the intima to the adventitia in the distal portion. In the proximal portion they suture the intima to the adventitia for half the circumference leaving a large reentrance for half the circumference. Death is usually due to external rupture. Half of the acute cases have their extent limited to the ascending aorta and arch of the aorta. The diagnosis of dissecting aneurysm by means of angiocardiography was first described by A Golden in 1949. A case of dissecting aneurysm of the aorta was diagnosed and the operated upon by Abbott. There was a fusiform enlargement of the aorta extending from just above the pericardial reflexion to 3 cm above the diaphragm. Seventy per cent was wrapped with cellophane and 5 months later the patient was doing well subjectively.

DeBakey and associates in 1956 reported on 13 patients on whom they had operated for an enlarged supracardiac shadow. Diagnosis was usually made after x-rays showed an enlarged supra cardiac shadow. About 90% of the patients with this condition will die within a few hours or weeks. If time permits an angiocardiogram will confirm the diagnosis. Surgical treatment may save the life of the patient but dissection may recur later. If the dissection starts in the ascending aorta and continues into the descending aorta the aorta is divided between clamps below the left subclavian artery. A small wedge shaped segment is excised from the dissected inner wall in the upper segment to create re-entry. The false passage is closed in the distal segment. The two segments are then reunited allowing blood to flow from the double lumen above into the single lumen below. The site of rentry is made as close to the beginning of the dissection as possible. The site of reentry is made as close to the beginning of the dissection as possible. If the dissection extends into the iliacs the procedure may be repeated just above the aortic bifurcation. If the intimal tear is at or distal to the left subclavian artery the involved aorta will have to be resected and replaced with a graft. The inner and outer walls of the distal segment must be sutured together. Ten of the thirteen patients they operated on recovered and have remained asymptomatic.

Warrren and Associates wrote about the management of a dissecting aneurysm of the aorta and reviewed some history. He wrote that in 1802 Maunoir was the first to publish a clear description of the condition. In 1882 Shekelton of Dublin lucidly described the distal opening through the intimal wall of the the sac. And pointed out the significance of the reopening from the aneurysm into the aorta. In 1855 the first clinical diagnosis of the condition was made by Swaine and associates and the diagnosis was confirmed at autopsy. From then until 1933 there were only five additional cases diagnosed before death. They suggested the possibility of creating a reentry site by partially occluding the aorta with a Satinsky clamp and then removing a small portion of the intima and then resuturing the aorta. This would make it possible to have the reentry site in the ascending aorta.

Bahnson and associates in 1956 reported a case of dissecting aneurysm of the aorta treated by fenestration. The basic pathological problem in dissecting aneurysm of the aorta is medial cystic necrosis. The cystic areas are connected by hematomas which form in the wall and extend along the wall usually entering the lumen through a tear in the wall. Blood under aortic pressure enters the wall and causes a more rapid dissection. When there is only one tear into the lumen It is possible for a second decompressing tear to occur spontaneously. Matas did much to advance our knowledge. His introduction of endoaneurysmoraphy was the first step towards a cure. However the curative surgery did not start until Dubost, in 1951 resected an abdominal aneurysm and replaced it with a homograft. After that DeBakey, and Bahnson and others attacked thoracic aortic aneurysms with success. Prefabricated grafts are now available for most if not all varieties of aneurysm and locations. This allows for branching at the brachiocephalic end or, the arch with the cervical and subclavian vessels. Dacron grafts are available in various shapes and sizes, enough to cover the various extent and locations of the aneurysm.

The gold standard of thoraco- abdominal aortic aneurysm has long been open surgical repair. Despite the technological advances in endo -vascular aortic repair open operation remains the preferred technique for these highly complex repairs. At experienced surgical centers the mortality for these procedures have greatly improved during the past 40 years even in patients with extensive repairs such as chronic aortic dissection or Marfan syndrome. Coselli reported an experience with 823 open thoracic and open abdominal repairs from Jan 2005 to May 2012, the 30 day mortality was 4.7% and the rate of permanent paraplegia was 3.8%. The mean age of this entire group was 63.4 years. The series included 75 emergent repairs (9.1%) 37 ruptured aneurysms (4.5%),322 chronic dissections (39.1%), and 264 Crawford extent 11 repairs (32.1) all of which are traditionally with the greatest risk of early death, spinal cord defect and renal failure. Within this series, 96 (11.7%) had connective-tissue disorders. Results were better in this subset (mean age 44.6) 91.6% of whom had had aortic dissection,- 83 with chronic aortic dissection (86.4%) and 5 with acute or subacute dissection(5.2%). The early mortality was 3.1% (3 patients)and the rate of permanent paraplegia was 1% (1patient). The rates of renal failure were similar in patients with connective tissue disorder (5.2%; 5 patients) and for patients without these disorders(5.5%; 45 patients)

These generally favorable results are being achieved despite the increasing complexity of TAAA surgery. These operations are increasingly being performed in elderly patients who have multiple comorbid conditions. Furthermore the growing popularity of endovascular thoracic aortic aneurysm repair has produced a group of patients who experience stent graft failure and require late conversion to open TAAA repair. There is a more frequent use of off label endovascular approaches in patients with chronic aortic dissection. In 2013 Nozdrzykowski and colleagues reported their experience treating chronic aortic dissection; nearly a quarter of patients who initially underwent endovascular repair experienced a severe complication (such as infection, rupture, new-onset paraplegia or a fistula) that ultimately required conversion to open surgery. Many of these were emergency conversions which inherently increase operative risk.

Their approach currently includes the selective use of several adjunctive techniques for organ protection such as left-sided heart bypass, cerebral spinal fluid drainage, selective visceral perfusion and cold renal perfusion. Prefabricated multibranched grafts can be used to separately reattach the visceral arterial branches thereby minimizing residual native aortic tissue. This is particularly important in patients with connective tissue disorders because it prevents the late formation of visceral patch aneurysms. In addition these mulibranched grafts shorten ischemic times and facilitate tension free anastomoses which might improve hemostasis and prevent late pseudoaneurysm formation.

This discussion of current results and adjunctive techniques for the surgeon gives a good update on current results with a consideration of the extent that bio- prostheses have taken over the surgical correction of aneurysms whether they be of arteriosclerotic, dissecting or connective tissue abnormality such as marfans syndrome. The mortality and complications have certainly come down to acceptable range considering the high mortalities and complications of the early struggles with these highly complex and dangerous entities.

Endovascular abdominal aneurysm results in more than 15,000 deaths annually the dangers in the chest are similar. In addition to the surgical procedures that we have described for the chest and abdomen for saccular or dissecting aneurysm there is another modality available in the bag of procedures for abdominal and even in select cases in the chest. The prehospitalization mortality rate of 59% to 83% and a mortality rate of 30to80% in patients who present for medical care gives you an idea of magnitude of the problem as well the risk treating these patients. The procedure is endovascular aneurysm repair with the use of endo grafts inserted through a femoral artery and positioned at the aneurysm. This procedure is a less invasive alternative, it avoids anesthesia, secures proximal control with the use of an aortic occlusion balloon, reduces blood loss, and avoids the need for open surgical procedure, rupture reports during the past two decades have cited lower 30 day mortality rates in EVAR (endovascular aneurysm repair) than in open repair.

The lessons of the past could aid our analysis of how to best manage patients with ruptured aortic aneurysm. Bahnson was the first to report the repair of a ruptured aortic aneurysm with a homograft in March 1953. The suprarenal extent of the aneurysm in that report would not have enabled the use of EVAR with the use of todays endographs. In 1954 Cooley and DeBakey published the first relevant case series. Three of six patients survived surgery for ruptured aortic aneurysm with the use of homografts. Cooley recommended expeditious repair and suprarenal aortic control just below the diaphragm over dissecting the hematoma in unstable patients. Preoperative transfusions were contraindicated because it raised the blood pressure and contributed to exsanguinating hemorrhage. The use of autotransfusion devices and non- porous Dacron grafts were recommended. Cooley's personal series at that time included 43 patients operated on for ruptured AAA with 36 survivors (84%). Crawford in 1991 focused on permissive hypotension and minimizing fluid resuscitation until the aorta was clamped. Hypotension was felt to be an important natural homeostatic mechanism that slowed bleeding and enabled clot formation. In Crawford's series of 87 patients with ruptured AAA 67 survived; 58% of patients with hypotension survived and 94% without hypotension survived. In the presence of cardiac arrest only 33% of patients survived. Of patients over 80, 73% survived.

Population-based studies that have used large United States data bases have shown a significantly reduced mortality for EVAR (30.4%-57.7%) versus open repair(40.7% -56.4%) In these studies EVAR was used in only 2.5% to 12% of patients. EVAR was used in only 2.5% to 12% of patients. Statistical differences in mortality rates were due to many factors and cannot be attributed to the procedure alone. In 2009 EVAR was used in 74% of elective AAA repairs but only 24% of ruptured AAA procedures. EVAR mortality rates in teaching hospitals was 21% versus 39% for open repair, however mortality rates for EVAR in non-teaching hospitals rose to 55% higher than for open repair (46%). The publication in 2013 of the results of the Amsterdam randomized trial gives some insight into the appropriate role of EVAR. 0f 520 patients with ruptured AAA who presented at 10 regional hospitals 11% died without treatment or during evaluation and 86 urgent surgeries were performed before unstable patients could undergo computed tomographic evaluation. Unfavorable anatomy for EVAR was present in 240 of 395 patients (60.8%)who underwent complete CT evaluation. 116 patients were ultimately randomized to EVAR or open repair at 3 treatment centers. Of the EVAR assigned patients 10 of 57 (17.5%) crossed over to surgery because of type 1 endo leak (5 patients) access failure (3 patients), cardiac arrest (1 patient) and lack of proper endograph (1 patient). In the randomized cohort the 30day mortality rate for EVAR was 21% versus 25% for open repair. In patients with unfavorable anatomy for EVAR the open- repair mortality was only 26%. In the hemodynamically unstable patients who underwent triage before CT scanning the data revealed an overall open-repair rate of was only 26%. In hemodynamically unstable patients who underwent triage before CT scanning the data revealed an overall open-repair mortality rate of 30%. The mortality rate was 38% for all 520 patients who presented with ruptured AAA. This randomized study yielded no significant difference in complication or mortality rates between EVAR and open repair. The lower than expected mortality rate in treated patients was attributed to optimization of logistics, preoperative CT imaging, and centralization of care. Conclusions are

- Patient selection bias restricts EVAR use in hemodynamically unstable patients who need immediate treatment
- Azizzadeh and colleagues reported that 83 patients who underwent open repair for ruptured AAA had an overall 30 day mortality of 21.4%. When cardiopulmonary resuscitation was applied the mortality rate was 100%.
- Hemodynamic instability worsened mortality rates (33% vs 18%)reduced the likelihood of a CT scan (64% vs 4%), necessitated an aortic balloon more often (40% vs 6%)and more often led to an abdominal compartment syndrome (29% vs 4%). The mortality rate in patients with abdominal compartment syndrome was 59%(vs 18% otherwise)
- In 2013 Dick and colleagues validated Crawford and Cooley's earlier observations by demonstrating the importance of delayed volume resuscitation during initial management of ruptured AAA. Preoperative fluid infusion correlated directly with 30 day mortality rates. Aggressive volume resuscitation should be delayed until bleeding is surgically controlled. The authors reported a 30 day mortality rate of 15% from open repair of ruptured AAA in 248 patients
- Another concern is that an EVAR- first strategy could delay definitive treatment. Time -to -death studies in untreated rupture patients showed a steep decline in survival rates: 40% to 50%of deaths occurred within 1 to 2 hours of emergent arrival.
- While CT imaging is helpful other studies have shown that delays in treatment increase mortality rates, prolong intensive care unit stays, and CT imaging might not be feasible for unstable patients.
- Studies have shown that CT images will reveal anatomy unsuitable for EVAR in up to 50% of patients because of aortic neck length, aortic diameter, or aortic neck angulation and iliac artery access.

In summary although EVAR has proved to be effective in selected patients with ruptured AAA it is not the treatment of choice for most patients. It could delay treatment and increase risk and delay treatment in hemodynamically unstable patients. Clinical trials showed no advantage in mortality or complication rates of EVAR versus open repair.

As a final note on endovascular aneurysm repair (EVAR) we must mention the report Galovitch et al who strongly recommend EVAR as a treatment option for elective aneurysm repair with lower short term morbidity and mortality rates. As physicians' comfort and confidence with the technique have increased EVAR has become the preferred treatment for ruptured infrarenal abdominal aortic aneurysm in their hands. Their claim is that since its inception in 1988 by Volodos endovascular repair of the aorta has been transformed. What began as an experimental procedure now accounts for most elective AAA repair. Ruptured endovascular aneurysm repair (rEVAR) has become the preferred treatment for many ruptured AAA's in centers that that have hybrid interventional rooms which can accommodate expedient open or endovascular repair. In comparison with open repair rEVAR has shown superior 30 day and 5 year mortality rates. Patients with ruptured AAA who are transferred for higher level of care have superior clinical outcomes when treated with rEVAR compared with open repair. One of the main arguments for performing rEVAR first is the high 30 day mortality rate associated with open repair (consistently near 50% vs around 25% for EVAR.)Even the 5 year rate for EVAR is better than that for open repair.(37% vs 26%). However there is still room for improvement, – especially with regard to the prevention and management of abdominal compartment syndrome. The principles for EVAR remain the same as for open repair, however the stent choice might vary from that for elective EVAR. After either femoral artery cutdown or percutaneous accesswire access is attained and a long sheath is placed to secure the position of a supraceliac aortic occlusion balloon in case it should be needed. The balloon should be inflated only for the purpose of providing hemodynamic stability because the use of aortic occlusion balloons is associated with abdominal compartment syndrome. Next intravascular ultrasound (IVUS) is used to evaluate the anatomy of the Aneurysm's neck and the access route for rEVAR. The IVUS can be used to confirm the computed tomographic (CT) findings or as the primary imaging technique in the absence of a preoperative CT. Although it makes sense to use that with which you are most familiar with, bear in mind that contralateral gate cannulation can prolong graft deployment- which should not be delayed. In rEVAR a unibody graft has the advantage in cases with difficult gate cannulation. Examples:an 85 year old woman with lower abdominal pain was found to have upon CT scanning a contained rupture of an AAA she underwent endovascular repair of the aneurysm with a unibody Endologix Endograft (Endologix, Irvine Calif). Patient 2: An 87 year old man with a history 12 years earlier of aorto/bifemoral bypass for a ruptured AAA presented with abdominal pain and was found to have a contained rupture of a para-anastamotic aortic aneurysm at the proximal suture line The ruptured para-anastomotic aneurysm was repaired by creating an aortic uni-iliac configuration – that is, a Talent Converterstent- graf system (Medtronic, Inc, Minneapolis, Minn) combined with an Endurant a aortic cuff (Medtronic, Inc) combined with a left to right femorofemoral bypass. No intervention has been required in the subsequent 2 year follow-up. Endovascular repair of ruptured aneurysm has a re-intervention rate of up to 20% with type 2 leaks being the most common indication. Their conclusion and experience are that the high mortality rate of the open repair could be improved by an EVAR first approach in centers that have hybrid intervential rooms which can accommodate expedient open or endovascular repair.

This illustrates an ongoing discussion as to the best approach to a very big problem much of which has to do with what the responsible group is comfortable with and perhaps what they are best equipted to do. There is one more item of interest that has recently surfaced and that is that routine screening is warranted for the first degree relatives who present with thoracic aortic disease before age 60 years in the absence of hypertension, Marfan's syndrome, or bicuspid aortic valve. Dr. Robertson of Royal Prince Alfred Hospital in Campertown, Australia, discovered that screening first degree relatives for familial thoracic aortic aneurysm is essential. They found two additional affected individuals on average per initial patient.

We have spent much of our discussion on aneurysms in general because there is a similarity in the pathology and the principles of treatment. The cystic medial necrosis, the dissection, the rupture, shape and size all play a role in the pathology and out come be it dissection without a leak, or dissection in the thorax involving the abdominal portion, rupture, shock, resuscitation, administration of blood, diagnostic procedures, the use of Dacron prostheses for ascending aorta, arch, descending, thoracic aorta, and aneurysms that involve the iliacs. All of these may be affected and there artificial grafts that will fit the needs of the surgeon and the patient. The principles outlined for the subdiaphragmatic aorta apply to the thoracic aorta. In the chest however there may be a need for a bypass circulation or even the heart lung machine if it involves the aortic valve.

CHAPTER 18

Chest Trauma

THE MORTALITY RATE in hospitalized patients with chest injuries is 4 to 8%. It is 10 to 15% when one other organ system is involved and rises to 35% when multiple organ systems are involved. With the design and development of high speed motor vehicles and motor cycles and now recreational vehicles such as light weight aircraft thoracic injuries are frequently encountered in the emergency setting. Although most of these are of minor magnitude and are not immediately life threatening autopsy studies have shown that a leading cause of on-site fatality is some type of injury involving the heart and great vessels. Of all blunt injuries to the chest 80% are caused by automobile accidents. Two of every three of these deaths occur after the patient reaches the hospital and can potentially be prevented with prompt diagnosis and correct management. Although 90% of chest injuries do not require thoracotomy immediate use of simple specific measures may be lifesaving. The immediate pathologic effect of most major thoracic injuries are tissue hypoxia and metabolic acidosis because of diminished cardiac output and pulmonary shunting. Hypoventilation, hypoxemia and respiratory acidosis and pulmonary shunting all are part of thoracic injury. Accurate diagnosis requires an assessment of those pathological states that may be immediately life threatening including airway obstruction massive hemothorax, cardiac tamponade, tension pneumoyhorax, flail chest, open pneumothorax, and massive tracheobronchial air leak. Patients with upper airway obstruction appear cyanotic, ashen or grey; there may be strident or gurgling sounds, ineffective respiratory excursions, and retraction of cervical, epigastric and, and intercostal muscles. If respiratory excursions are not visible ventilation is probably inadequate. Paradoxical chest wall movement in flail chest is usually located anteriorly and can generally be visualized. Sucking chest wounds are obvious. A large hemothorax can usually be detected by percussion and subcutaneous emphysema is easily detected by palpation. Both massive hemothorax and tension pneumothorax can easily be detected by diminished breath sounds and a shift of the trachea to the contralateral side. If the patient has an absent or thready pulse and distended neck veins the main differential diagnosis is between cardiac tamponade and tension pneumothorax. In moribund patients immediate treatment is chest tube placement, pericardiocentesis, or thoracotomy. An adequate airway must be established and effective ventilation must be demonstrated. The 3 leading causes of in ineffective ventilation after establishing an endotracheal tube are collapse of the lung by either air or blood or mal position of the endotracheal tube. These three factors must be excluded following successful intubation of the patient whether it be blunt or penetrating. Evaluation of the circulation whether it be blunt or penetrating will identify patients with a cardiac injury leading to tamponade.

Rib fracture may be the most common injury. Localized pain and tenderness and crepitus will make the diagnosis. A chest x-ray is needed to exclude other intrathoracic injuries and not necessarily to identify rib fracture. Narcotics in small amounts and intercostal nerve blocks usually suffice for the fractured rib. Cough assistance and endotracheal suction for several days may be necessary. Fracture of the upper ribs, clavicle and or scapula usually indicate significant trauma.

Unilateral fracture of four or five ribs will produce enough instability that paradoxical respiratory motion results in hypoventilation of an unacceptable degree. Although usually not apparent in the conscious patient it is usually visible in the unconscious patient. If severe and untreated atelectasis and hypercapnea, hypoxia and accumulation of secretions and ineffective cough occur. These pathophysiological findings may be present immediately or may progress over several hours and present as late respiratory decompensation. Certain combinations of rib fracture and sternal fracture may be bad enough to warrant open reduction. At this time endotracheal intubation with the use of a volume respirator is indicated. A respiratory rate greater than 40 and a po2 less than 60 on 60% FIO2 are indications for intubation. In addition pre- existing chronic lung disease, depressed level of consciousness and concomitant abdominal injuries are relative indications. Once the patient has been ventilated the use of serial intercostal blocks of the ribs or even a segmental epidural block, may be helpful in reducing pain and hypoventilation. In addition almost 100% of the patients with a flail chest have a significant underlying pulmonary contusion that will contribute to the hypoxia secondary to intra parenchymal shunting. An awareness of this contribution is necessary in determining whether or not positive end expiratory pressure (PEEP) is necessary for treatment. Trinkle and associates point out that that the need for ventilation assistance may be reduced and that parenchymal contusion is the more significant lesion. Sucking wounds of the chest (open pneumothorax), a defect in the chest wall with an opening that allows air to suck in and be expelled without ventilation of the lung on the affected side may produce complete collapse of the lung unless ventilation with an endotracheal tube is in place. The resultant shift of the mediastinum and diminished cardiac output can be life threatening. Treatment consists of closure of the wound with a sterile dressing and continuous evacuation of the pleural space with a chest tube and underwater seal to prevent tension pneumothorax.

Critical intrathoracic injury in the form of pulmonary contusion can occur in the absence of rib fracture. This is especially important in children whose rib cage is very elastic. Fluid and blood from ruptured vessels enter the alveoli and interstitial spaces and bronchi and produce respiratory obstruction. Pulmonary contusion may produce a localized hematomas and may be confused with adult respiratory syndrome (ARDS). X-ray examination will show the consolidation from minimal to lobar.

MANAGEMENT involves careful ventilator support and effective clearing of secretions. Fluid should be administered with care so as not to overload and albumin may be hepful to maintain osmotic pressure of the blood. Hemmorhage and edema are self limited and will clear if infection is avoided. Positive-end-- expiratory- pressure (PEEP) may be a useful adjunct in the management of these patients.

Pneumothorax: this occurs with laceration of the lung via rib fracture or rupture of alveoli following penetrating or blunt trauma. Tension pneumothorax occurs when a flap valve leak occurs and allows air to enter the pleural space but does not allow the escape of air. Intra- pleural pressure rises causing total lung collapse and a shift of the mediastinum to the other side. This pressure must be relieved immediately to avoid interference with ventilation of the opposite lung. It may also interfere with return of venous blood to the heart. Tension pneumothorax is is a true surgical emergency requiring immediate diagnosis and decompression by a chest tube and under water seal. In most cases water seal suction is all that is needed. The temptation to watch a pneumothorax should be avoided. The possibility of a pneumothorax developing into a true emergency when the patient is transferred to the ward must always be considered. It should be documented by chest x-ray.

HEMORRHAGE INTO THE PLEURAL SPACE. This occurs in almost every patient with a diagnosable chest injury. Blood loss can vary from slight to extensive. As much as 300 to 500 cc of blood may be present and not noticed in a chest xray done in the supine position Bleeding may be from any organ in the chest such as the heart or great vessels. Most often it is from the intercostal vessels or even the internal mammary artery in sternal injuries. Early tube thoracostomy with a no. 30 F chest tube will prevent late fibrothorax. With massive hemothorax the blood can be collected for autotransfusion. In 85% of the patients tube thoracostomy is the treatment that is required immediately. Thoracotomy is reserved for those with a massive hemothorax which in almost every case will reveal the source of bleeding. Signs of persisting bleeding such as 1500cc will also indicate exploratory thoracotomy.

TRACHEAL AND BRONCHIAL INJURIES:Blunt tracheal or bronchial injuries are often due to compression of the airways between sternum and vertebral column as in decelerating steering wheel accidents. With tracheal injuries patients present with tracheal or laryngeal crepitus, subcutaneous emphysema, hoarseness, and evolving airway obstruction. When accompanied by acute airway obstruction the immediate priority is the establishment of an effective airway. If an endoscopic exam can be done this should precede the placement of an endotracheal tube. If an endotracheal tube cannot be passed and endoscopy cannot be done, tracheostomy is indicated. More commonly the distal trachea or mainstem bronchus is involved and such patients present with hemo-pneumothorax, subcutaneous emphysema, pneumomediastinum, hemoptysis and airway obstruction. When early diagnosis is made the contralateral bronchus is intubated and the primary repair is performed. However when a partial or complete stricture results bronchiectasis and parenchymal destruction results. If an early stricture results resection and repair can be done. However if parenchymal destruction of the lung has occurred the resection is the only option. Penetrating injuries of the diaphragm outnumber blunt injuries. However small wounds such as a knife wound can result in herniation of lung. Such herniations may be found years later. Most herniations from blunt trauma usually follow automobile accidents and may involve any part of the diaphragm often radial in configuration. Herniation may not occur immediately and may escape immediate diagnosis. On the left side herniation may not occur immediately or may not be noticed because of the injuries to abdominal organs that require treatment. On the right side diaphragm injuries may not be noticeable. CT and liver scans are helpful in ruling out right diaphragm injuries. With injuries on the left side of the diaphragm the surgical approach is best through the abdomen; on the right side it may be necessary to approach it through a right thoracotomy.

HEART AND PERICARDIUM

Blunt injury to the heart usually occurs from compression by the steering column. The injury may vary from a contusion of the heart to actual rupture. Fifty percent of autopsies performed on victims of automobile accidents show damage to the heart and pericardium. Myocardial damage may vary from petechiae to transmural damage and actual bleeding usually damage to the right ventricle which can occur at the time of the accident to delayed bleeding from the heart Injury and thrombosis of the coronary vessels can result from this type of injury. Although most patients with this type of injury never get to the hospital, some with tears of atrium or vena cava do reach the hospital. Rupture of the interventricular septum has been reported and results in a large left to right shunt. Early signs include friction rubs chest pain, murmurs, arrhythmias and evidence of low cardiac output. Electrocardiograms will show non-specific ST and T wave changes. Intensive Care monitoring is indicated if there are EKG changes. Echocardiography may be helpful in diagnosing dysfunction of the ventricular wall. The management of myocardial contusion should be the same that for myocardial infarction.

TAMPONADE

Tamponade in blunt cardiac trauma is uncommon and when it does it is due to myocardial rupture or coronary artery laceration. Penetrating trauma with myocardial injury is the most common cause and is easily diagnosed. Tamponade of relatively small amounts of blood will produce distended neck veins, shock and cyanosis. Immediate treatment is pericardiocentesis which will also give you the diagnosis. When available echocardiography is helpful in making a diagnosis. Hemothorax, shock and exsanguination occur in cases of gunshot wounds. Gunshot wounds are less likely than stab wounds to present as tamponade. Prompt thoracotomy with decompression of the tamponade and suture of the bleeding site are indicated. The presence of a post injury cardiac murmur will probably require cardiac catheterization and perhaps a valve replacement or repair of aseptal defect.

AORTA INJURY

Injury of the thoracic aorta are seen with increasing frequency. The mechanism of injury is not fully understood but it is thought that the aortic arch at the beginning of the descending aorta undergoes flexion or torsion disrupting the aortic wall at the ligamentum arteriosum immediately distal to the subclavian artery. Occasionally the ascending aorta at its root is injured or several intercostal arteries are severed. Most patients with aortic rupture die immediately. However about 20% will be able to contain the blood loss producing a traumatic aneurysm. Typically there is partial or complete circumferential tear. Those who survive the initial tear develop a false aneurysm which will slowly enlarge over the years. Other lesions such as intracranial trauma, chest wall injury, or ruptured spleen may explain the clinical findings. The most common finding may be a widening of the mediastinum on chest xray with loss of the aortic contour, shift of the endotracheal tube and trachea to the right elevation of the left mainstem bronchus, depression of the right main stem bronchus, shift of the nasogastric tube to the left, apical capping, first rib fracture, acute left sided hemothorax, and retro cardiac density. Retrograde aortography is the standard for diagnosis. Surgical care should be performed immediately. A shunt or bypass may be required. Several methods of byass have been used with the aim of protecting the spinal cord. A Teflon or Dacron graft will probably be needed if end-to-end repair cannot be done.

ESOPHAGUS

Blunt injuries to the esophagus are rare. The most common symptom of esophageal perforation is extreme pain followed by fever perhaps regurgitation of blood, perhaps hoarseness, dysphagia, or respiratory distress. X-rays may show a foreign body, perhaps air in the mediastinum, dysphagia and even respiratory distress if there is injury to the trachea. X-rays may also show mediastinal air or hydro-pneumomediastinum. The most common form of esophageal injury follows penetrating trauma but it can happen at esophagoscopy if the patient is not well sedated or under general anesthesia. One of the most surprising finding is a foreign body like a whole dental prosthesis.

Esophageal injury or the suspicion of perforation requires x-rays, esophagoscopy if it has not already been done, immediate debridement and suture closure.

CHAPTER 19

Pulmonary Embolism

PULMONARY EMBOLISM IS a significant complication of a number of medical and surgical disorders as well as such mundane activities as travel in a car or airplane usually for long distances. Detailed studies of the lung on routine postmortem examinations reveal a high incidence of pulmonary embolism especially in patients over age 40. At first the thrombus in the pulmonary artery arose in the pulmonary artery. It was Rudolf Virchow, around 1846, who convincingly demonstrated the embolic origin of clots in the lungs. Patients with pulmonary emboli were shown to have associated venous thrombi in their legs and pelvis as a source. Virchow was able to differentiate the clots that originated from the legs or pelvis to the clots in the lungs that were secondary to the local pulmonary clots resulting secondary to stasis produced by embolic clots. Usually both lungs are affected. The ultimate effect of massive pulmonary embolus is sudden death. Survivors may show spontaneous regression with a return to normal function in several weeks provided that no more clots find their way to the lungs. Pulmonary emboli may occur in children also though the incidence of pulmonary emboli is higher in the elderly (>than 54 years) with an appreciable incidence of underlying cardiac and pulmonary disease. There is significant experimental data that shows that shutting off circulation to one lung is well tolerated by most individuals. However with massive pulmonary emboli both lungs are usually affected. Pulmonary artery pressure may be increased 12-50% while cardiac output may increase as much as three fold. Hypoxemia and peripheral cyanosis are known to be manifestations of severe pulmonary embolism. Clinical evidence of reflex broncho-constriction has been described. Intravenous heparin has been shown to improve pulmonary function. Humoral factors mediated by platelets may be important in the genesis of cardiopulmonary disturbances. Recurrent pulmonary embolism may be a cause of chronic heart disease. It has been termed "primary pulmonary hypertension". Clinical manifestation could be more or less characteristic of pulmonary embolism including the respiratory symptoms and repeated episodes but the other group consists of patients without any radiologic evidence or gross pulmonary event in whom the condition is first recognized in the advanced stages. Pulmonary arteriography is especially helpful in diagnosing these patients. It is estimated that approximately 50,000 deaths occur each year in the United States as a result of pulmonary embolism. The risk of mortality from pulmonary embolism following surgical procedures in 1954 (DeBakey) in a collected series of pulmonary embolism was found to be .11 per cent. Several European studies have shown a rise in the incidence during the course of the study. In the Oxford study the incidence rose 5x during the course of the study and approximately half were fatal. The characteristic dyspnea, chest pain, hemoptysis, and hypertension may be present but are not specific. Additional findings include tachycardia, accentuation of the second pulmonary sound, dilation of the cervical veins and an enlarged, pulsating liver. The classic signs of dyspnea and tachypnea are the most frequent clinical findings. Hemoptysis, pleural friction, gallop rhythm, cyanosis and chest splinting are present in only a quarter or less of patients. Clinical evidence of phlebitis occurs in only a third of the patients. The plain chest film may only show diminished pulmonary vascular markings. Physical signs and plain chest x-ray are frequently insufficient to establish a diagnosis. Serum enzymes and bilirubin may be elevated but are non-specific. The EKG may be helpful but again is non- specific. Wagner in 1964 did radio-isotope pulmonary scanning. It thus possible to delineate the distribution of pulmonary arterial blood flow and reveal areas of under perfusion. Pathologic lesions of the lung may also show under perfusion and need to be excluded from consideration. Pulmonary angiography is an excellent technique for demonstration of the patency of these vessels. If arteriography is performed later in the course of this disease the findings may be a little confusing, the contrast medium may pass around the obstruction.

Management of pulmonary embolism: Anticoagulation is the primary form of treatment. In the acute stages intravenous heparin drip is an effective means to maintain clotting time at twice normal. This may be followed by prophylactic coumadin anticoagulation though this carries some increased hazard in the elderly population. A number of surgical interventions have been proposed and used effectively over the past half century. We will mention them but it is important to realize that there is no perfect or universally successful or safe technique. Interruption of the inferior vena cava by ligation or plication techniques have been advocated by a number authors. Greenfield and associates have designed a cone shaped steel device designed to trap emboli without significant reduction in venous flow. This filter may be inserted under local anesthesia through in either the jugular or femoral vein. Distal migration of this filter down to the bifurcation of the vena cava has occurred and the struts have also protruded through the caval wall. In Greenfield's series recurrent embolism rate was 3% and the mortality was 4%. The Greenfield filter is less likely to promote thrombosis in the inferior vena cava than the filter designed by Mobin-Uddin. In males the inferior vena cava is preferably approached through a flank incision on the right side and in females it is preferable to approach the vena cava through an abdominal incision in order to expose and ligate the ovarian veins. Direct venous thrombectomy was described by Mahorner et al (1957) to reduce and prevent chronic venous insufficiency and also to prevent or reduce the likelihood of pulmonary embolism. Favorable results have been reported however others warned of a high incidence of postthrombectomy thrombosis. Massive pulmonary embolism and shock have occurred during the course of ileofemoral thrombectomy. Most advocates of this procedure recommend immediate anticoagulation with heparin and its continued use postoperatively to prevent recurrent thrombosis.

For the patient in pulmonary and cardiac distress the procedures described above are not a solution. Now we have the option of doing a direct thrombectomy on the pulmonary artery using extracorporeal heart-lung circulation with or without hypothermia. The first attempt to remove massive emboli from the pulmonary artery was by Trendelenburg (1908) in three patients but in each the procedure ended fatally. And Kirchner (1924) a student of Trendelenburg was the first to perform a successful pulmonary embolectomy. The first successful pulmonary embolectomy in the United States was reported by Steenberg et al (1958). In the days before open heart operations the chest is entered as an emergency procedure, the pulmonary artery is opened and the emboli are removed. There is little doubt that more patients died as a result of Trendelenberg operations than survived them. The first successful removal of pulmonary emboli with temporary occlusion of the circulation and hypothermia to 29 degrees was reported from Oxford University in 1960 (Allison et al). The ideal method is to use cardiopulmonary bypass and this was reported by Sharp in 1962 and since then a number of surgeons have reported their results.

The results of a cooperative survey of cardiovascular surgeons in the US and Canada were reported by Cross and Mowlem (1967). The study evaluates 137 patients of whom 115 had the procedure with cardiopulmonary bypass. Thrombi were found in both pulmonary arteries in 110 patients (72%). Of the 7 patients in whom no thrombi were found at operation all succumbed following operation. This emphasizes the need for accurate diagnosis. The time that elapses between onset of symptoms and death is important since it is related to the time associated with preparation for an operative procedure. An analysis of results divided the patients into two groups: those who were in good general condition and those with terminal illnesses. In the first group 55% lived longer than two hours and 48% actually lived eight hours or longer. In the terminally ill patients only 32% survived longer than 2 hours. Thus in the group without terminal illness, more than half survived long enough to allow for preparation for extracorporeal circulation and direct embolectomy. The operation may be performed with opening either the right or left chest the side with the greater involvement usually being selected. In properly selected patients chronic pulmonary embolism may be managed successfully by embolectomy. Routine chest films, radioactive scans, and angiography, and pulmonary function testing should be available for proper selection of patients.

EPILOGUE

THIS HAS BEEN a bit of medical about what is possible in Thoracic (chest) surgery which includes the surgical treatment of some of the most important organs of everyone's existence. We have attempted to review some of the most spectacular achievements in the history of surgery in the last 100 years though most have occurred in the last 60 years and especially since 1948 when heart surgery really began with the living triumphs of such persistent stalwarts as Dwight Harken MD and Charles Bailey who first attacked the problem of rheumatic heart disease with their initial successes to correct mitral stenosis and thence onto the more difficult valve diseases of mitral insufficiency, aortic stenosis and aortic insufficiency. This can only be described as a beginning of a world wide effort to cure all forms of heart disease. There were earlier successes in the treatment of lung disease but much depended on the availability of antibiotics which did finally arrive by World War II which by the way gave Dr. Harken the opportunity to operate on live patients to remove foreign bodies from the heart and thus gain invaluable experience. The removal of an entire lung and also parts of lungs takes us back to the 1930s but this too evolved from a situation of unacceptable risk to life to a daily occurrence in the treatment of cancer and tuberculosis. I do not propose that I have covered every advance made or every pioneer that contributed to the vast number of operations devised and done by the pioneers and the many patients who benefited from their tireless efforts. I can appreciate their acomplishments because I was there, operated with them, and experienced some of the drama of bringing forth something new, meeting the world leaders, and in some small way participated on a daily basis either in the operating room or in the dog laboratory. In most descriptions I did not include the technical details of the operation but have tried to give you a fair assessment of what was accomplished and the results. There were failures and deaths along the way but we must also remember that the early efforts dealt with the sickest of the sick and with children as well as the elderly who had no future except the new operations and these gave the sick of the world optimism and life.

ACHNOWLEDGEMENTS

THE MATERIAL IN this book was obtained from a large number of sources and authors to include personal material; personal experience; personal conversations; published papers; numerous text books; medical and surgical journals published by medical and surgical societies; The Practice of Surgery (Harper and Rowe Publishers, 1978); 100 Years of Surgical Quality Improvement (American College of Surgeons); The Future of Surgical Simulation and Surgical Robotics (American College of Surgeons, March 2007); The Future of Robotics, Bulletin, (American College of Surgeons, July 2013); Texas Heart Institute Journal; Wikipedia; Science Week. Com; Thoracic Surgery News; Textbook of Surgery, Thirteenth Edition, Edited by David C Sabiston, Jr, MD,1986; A History of Thoracic Surgery, Edited by Richard H. Meade, MD, 1961; Thoracic Surgery and Related Pathology, Edited by Gustaf E Lindskog, MD, and Averill A Liebow, MD; Surgery of the Chest, Edited by John H Gibbon, Jr, MD, David C Sabiston, Jr, MD, Frank C Spencer, MD, second edition, 1969; Rapid Interpretation of EKG's, third edition, Dale Dubin, MD, 1975.

ABOUT THE AUTHOR

THE AUTHOR IS Armand A. Lefemine, MD, from Harvard Medical School (1952). His internship was at US Public Health hospital, and his surgical residency at VA Hospital, in Boston. This was followed by his fellowship with Dwight Harken, MD, in cardiac and thoracic surgery and his appointments at Harvard Medical School and Peter Bent Brigham Hospital. Then he had his private practice of thoracic and cardiac surgery in Hartford, Connecticut, and St. Elizabeth's Hospital in Boston, Massachusetts. He was faculty of Tufts Medical School, in Boston, Massachusetts. He was chief of surgery at VA Hospital in Johnson City, Tennessee and a professor of surgery at ETSU Medical School. He was chairman of the department of surgery at ETSU medical school, in Johnson City, Tennessee, and director of surgery for the Veterans Administration in Washington, DC.

www.ingramcontent.com/pod-product-compliance
Lightning Source LLC
Chambersburg PA
CBHW030924180526
45163CB00002B/460